COKE

COKE

THE BIOGRAPHY

NATALIA NAISH & JEREMY SCOTT

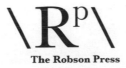

The Robson Press

First published in Great Britain in 2013 by
The Robson Press (an imprint of Biteback Publishing Ltd)
Westminster Tower
3 Albert Embankment
London SE1 7SP

ISBN 978-1-84954-517-4

10 9 8 7 6 5 4 3 2 1

A CIP catalogue record for this book is available from the British Library.

Set in Chronicle

Printed and bound in Great Britain by
CPI Group (UK) Ltd, Croydon CR0 4YY

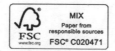

That sunny dome! those caves of ice!

And all who heard should see them there,

And all should cry, Beware! Beware!

His flashing eyes, his floating hair!

Weave a circle round him thrice,

And close your eyes with holy dread,

For he on honey-dew hath fed,

And drunk the milk of Paradise.

'Kubla Khan', Samuel Taylor Coleridge, 1797

CONTENTS

INTRODUCTION

HANS RAUSING (1963–) PART I

It was only urgent need for cash that got Hans Rausing out of bed that afternoon. He and his wife had been using heavily since the night before, Eva particularly so. They were almost out of gear.

Hans needed a hit to get himself together. Taking up the pipe, the bowl covered with perforated foil, he set it to his lips. With his right hand he snapped on the lighter and directed its jet of flame on the small rock of crack cocaine balanced on the silver paper. He inhaled deeply, drawing the sweet vapour into his lungs.

Within seconds his heartbeat soared, his head cleared and delusive vigour together with a ghost of will returned to him. This gave him the strength to pass the pipe to Eva, swing his legs to the floor and stand up. He started for the bathroom, picking his way through a litter of discarded syringes, charred scraps of foil and bloodied tissues. The two rooms the couple lived in had not been cleaned for months and the place looked like a squat.

The bedroom, with fetid air trapped within shut windows and curtains that remained drawn all day to exclude the sun, gave off the characteristic reek of the worst kind of crack den; the smell of unwashed bodies, stale tobacco and soiled sheets.

What was incongruous about this particular crack den was its location. The Rausings' six-storey house in Cadogan Place was worth £70 million and their fortune was estimated at £4 billion. This was serious money, even in London's Belgravia, which is colonised by Russian oligarchs, Arab princes and the cream of international non-doms. Many of them may be dodgy, but they are all part of the global super-rich.

Leaving the bathroom door ajar, Hans went to the mirror to shave. Stubble darkened his jaw and cheeks in a face that had grown gaunt and cadaverous. Neither of them had eaten for some time. He could have called the Filipino staff who left them meals on a tray at the foot of the stairs – the servants were banned from ascending onto the second floor. But neither Hans nor Eva had any appetite.

Lathering his face, Hans started to shave with a shaky hand. His concentration was focused. The hit he'd taken would last no longer than ten minutes, enough to clean up and get dressed. He'd need another in order to leave the house, get to the cash machine in Sloane Square 250 yards away and make it home. Then he'd call the Man...

He'd completed one side of his face, whose flesh had been denied sunlight for so long that it showed pallid white below lank unwashed hair. He looked like a vagrant. As he put the razor to the other cheek, the sound of a thump came from the room behind him.

I heard Eva slide off the bed. I went to the bedroom and saw her sitting on the floor. She was leaning sideways and her face was resting on a pillow. I heard her exhale and then she did not move at all. I saw her alive for just a few seconds. I went to her and grabbed her and tried to pull her up. I remember shouting, 'Eva, Eva, Eva' and turned her toward me and saw her eyes had dimmed. She had stopped breathing before I reached her. I knew she was dead...

She was still clutching the crack pipe in her hand.

Months later Hans would say he had no memory of what happened next but 'with the benefit of hindsight I think I did not act rationally. I sat with her for a period of time then covered her up with a blanket and duvet.' He had difficulty detaching the pipe from her clenched fingers because her grip was so tight. 'I couldn't look at her. I could not cope with her dying and do not feel able to cope with the reality of her death...'

Earlier that year Eva had gone to rehab in California – the last of countless similar attempts – and checked out early to come home to him. She had been absent only for a few days but he'd struggled to get by without her support. They were unable to communicate or relate to others and had severed their social connection with the world – and quite a privileged one it had been. Their circle included the Prince of Wales and Camilla. Hans and Eva were alone in the dependency they shared.

He had to protect her, Hans reasoned with a cracked and faulty brain. What followed took time, and more than once he had need of a hit to continue. He went to the large linen cupboard on the landing by their bedroom. Raking out the contents of the bottom shelf, he created a snug and private space. He wrapped her body in as many duvets as he could find and rolled the bundle onto the shelf. He locked the door.

It wasn't until the fourth day that he noticed the smell leaking from the closet. He found a can of deodoriser and sprayed the bundle till it was soaked and relocked the door. It was warm in the linen cupboard and three days later the smell of putrescence was back.

In the kitchen Hans found another can of air freshener and a roll of tape. He opened the closet and dragged out the bundle, wrapped it in plastic bin bags and secured it with string. His actions were methodical, deliberate and performed with an underwater slowness. He was not smoking crack now but mainlining heroin, which dulled the anguish and dread that was always present.

He manoeuvred the unwieldy package back into the closet. Locking the door, he sealed its edges with gaffer tape. Returning to the bedroom he knotted a tie around his upper arm, took up a syringe, probed for a main vein, shot up some smack and resumed his vigil...

AND GOD CREATED COKE

THE TREE OF LIFE

It's a nondescript rangy-looking plant with small white flowers and nothing distinctive about it except its insatiable urge to grow and flourish. When cultivated and pruned, its abundant leaves can be harvested four times a year.

The Tree of Life – that is how the coca bush was named and venerated in pre-Columbian South America. Viewed from where we stand today, the label appears spurious, even fatally misleading.

In the sixteenth century, Spanish explorers noted the indigenous peoples' habit of chewing coca leaves. To this day, the custom has not changed, and the modern *coquero* still stores the leaves in a wad in his cheek. The wad is then poked with a stick he has dipped into the *iscupuru*, a bag containing burnt roots, smashed seashells, lime or ash to release the alkaloids in the coca and produce a subtle high.

At first the *coquero*'s saliva turns green and his cheeks go numb. Then he begins to feel its effects: he is no longer hungry, though his stomach is empty. Strength, energy and optimism return to him. The lack of oxygen in the high Andes and the harshness of his life become more bearable.

Coca can be chewed or brewed and drunk as a tea. It does not appear to be either addictive or harmful and is used to cure altitude sickness or supplement an inadequate diet with essential nutrients and vitamins. Were it not for one aspect, the coca plant might be thought of as little more than a mild stimulant comparable to chocolate or coffee. But the leaf's 1 per cent cocaine content changes everything and has transformed it into one of the most expensive and controversial commodities in the world.

CREATION MYTHS

Coca has been venerated by South Americans for thousands, if not tens of thousands of years. Coca found in burial sites from 3000 BC and ancient clay figures with bulging cheeks attest to the constancy of the habit. The word coca is derived from Amyara, a pre-Incan language. The Incas built upon creation myths of earlier cultures to develop a rich folklore of death and regeneration centring on coca. In one legend, a coca plant springs out of the grave of a woman who has been dismembered for her rampant promiscuity. Another tale features the universal tropes of flood and regeneration with an added twist. The god Khuno punishes the Altiplano Indians by unleashing a storm which destroys their jungle homeland. Amidst the wreckage there is a single coca plant, and after consuming it, they find the strength to rebuild their lives.

Coca played both a spiritual and practical role in maintaining the Inca Empire, which, at its height (c. 1438–1533), spanned 75 per cent of the west coast of South America.

Paved roads allowed for rapid communication by relay messengers, who used coca to sustain them on their long-distance runs. Without a writing system, *quipus* or knotted strings made of llama hair were used to record events. They were deciphered by coca-chewing sages.

Because of coca's anaesthetising properties it was administered to those about to be sacrificed or trepanned. The divine plant was usually restricted to royal personages, court orators and priests, who offered it to the gods and conjured spirits with it during religious ceremonies. One wonders if their compulsory congregation, denied access to the cup, experienced quite the same exalted visions.

A DISGUSTING HABIT

Early in the conquest of the New World, Spanish explorers looked on the phenomenon of coca chewing with bemusement or revulsion. In 1504 Amerigo Vespucci notes: 'They all had their cheeks swollen out with a green herb inside, which they were constantly chewing like beasts, so they could scarcely utter speech, we were unable to comprehend their secret, nor with what object they acted thus.' By the time Pizarro finished off the Inca Empire in the late 1530s with the help of European weaponry and diseases, he and his cohorts hoped the plant might generate income as a cash crop. The Europeans did not take to it.

The problem was not the product's quality but its image. Mastication was unaesthetic and uncivilised. How could you look decent or even speak properly with a wad of coca in your cheek? Besides, they dismissed its supposed qualities as primitive hallucinations.

Without obvious monetary reward to be gained from coca, the Catholic Church, bent on stamping out any vestigial barbarism amongst the natives, anathematised it: 'The plant is idolatry and the work of the Devil, and appears to give strength only by a deception of the Evil One.' The matter was brought up at the First and Second Councils of Lima in 1552 and 1569. In a span of only four years, Don Francisco de Toledo, Viceroy of Peru, issued seventy ordinances against it. But coca was never actually *banned*, because the Indians, who were relied upon for the essential task of unearthing silver to ship back to Spain, absolutely refused to work without it. As usual, economics trumped religious scruples.

Coca was grudgingly condoned because it helped the Indians (who requested coca instead of payment because they distrusted European currency) to endure the toxic conditions in the mines. De Toledo introduced a labour tax or *mita*, which required all men to work in the mines for up to four months of the year and was, in effect, a form of slavery. Tens of thousands of Indians died from exhaustion and poisoning, receiving nothing but coca leaves in recompense.

DISCOVERY

Unlike other New World crops such as tobacco and cacao, coca was essentially ignored by Europeans until the eighteenth century. There are a few early references to it, including the 1662 poem 'A Legend of Coca' by Abraham Cowley, and a detailed description of the plant by a doctor from Seville. In 1735, the French botanist Joseph de Jussieu brought some leaves back to the Museum of Natural History where they were examined by the scientist Carl Linnaeus. The *Erythroxylum coca* species was belatedly classified in 1786.

On his 1801 expedition to Peru, the explorer Alexander von Humboldt expressed an interest in coca but mistakenly attributed its uplifting effects to the lime the Indians kept in their *iscupuru*. Another German determined 'that the moderate use of coca is not merely innocuous, but that it may be very conducive to the health'. Others violently disagreed with him and, from early on, public opinion on coca and then cocaine was divided.

In the 1800s, scientists began isolating nitrogen-based compounds in plants, known as alkaloids, which seemed to hold endless medical and commercial possibilities. Morphine was extracted from opium in 1803, quinine and caffeine were isolated in 1829 and nicotine in 1833. It was only a matter of time before cocaine was isolated from coca.

The main impediment to the research was meagre supplies of healthy leaves because they travelled badly. In 1857, chemist Friedrich Wöhler asked scientist Carl Scherzer who was travelling on Franz Josef's ship *Novara*, to collect as many coca leaves as possible on his journey to South America. When Scherzer returned in 1859 with 14 kilos, work could begin. Wöhler assigned the project to his brilliant PhD student, Albert Niemann, who took two years to isolate the coca alkaloid successfully. The 26-year-old published his seminal dissertation, *On a New Organic Base in the Coca Leaves*, in 1860 but died shortly after handing it in. Wilhelm Lossen took over the project, arriving at cocaine's chemical formula in 1863.

Niemann's steps for producing cocaine were relatively straightforward. First he soaked the leaves in a solution of alcohol and sulphuric acid. After draining the liquid, he was left with a sticky substance to which he added bicarbonate of soda. He then distilled the mixture with ether and was left with a pile of white crystals. Niemann followed the same nomenclature of nicotine, morphine and other alkaloids by naming his product coca-ine or cocaine. And so was born the drug of our title.

WHAT IS IT?

Cocaine ($C_{17}H_{21}NO_4$) is a crystalline alkaloid. In its hard salt form (hydrochloride), it is ground into powder, mixed with other substances and usually snorted (it can also be consumed orally, vaginally etc.) or dissolved in water and injected. Cocaine hydrochloride cannot be smoked because its melting point is too high. Crack cocaine, which is yellow-ish to brown rather than white, is the base form of powdered cocaine. It is not water soluble and can be smoked because it vaporises at 90 degrees rather than 190 degrees.

Cocaine is a central nervous stimulant that, like coffee, is an appetite suppressant. It also acts as a local anaesthetic. It constricts the blood vessels and increases body temperature, blood pressure and heart rate. Its effects are subtle rather than overpowering which is why it took doctors some time to cotton on to the fact that it can be harmful and addictive – both physically and psychologically.

Unlike heroin, which is rarely taken casually, some people are able to use cocaine recreationally without it negatively impacting their lives. Others become hopelessly hooked.

Excessive use can lead to heart attacks and various health problems. Cocaine deaths are rare – unless combined with heroin as a speedball – but not impossible.

A cocaine high doesn't last very long – about thirty minutes for powder and even less for crack. The reason it makes users feel good is because it blocks the re-uptake function of several neurotransmitters including dopamine, serotonin and norepinephrine. Instead of being reabsorbed, they accumulate in the nerve synapses and flood the user with feelings of energy and well-being. Dopamine is the chemical that is most associated with the body's reward system and is released when we eat, have sex or take drugs. With extended cocaine use, the dopamine receptors are killed off and it takes stronger and stronger doses to work.

AN EARLY FAN

Paolo Mantegazza was an Italian doctor who became entranced with the coca leaf shortly before Niemann synthesised cocaine. After experimenting on himself in 1859, he penned a rapturous paean to coca:

God is unjust because he made man incapable of sustaining the effects of coca lifelong. I prefer a life of ten years with coca to one of a hundred thousand without it. It seemed to me that I was separated from the whole world, and I beheld the strangest images, most beautiful in colour and in form, that can be imagined.

Mantagazza was amongst the first to believe that coca could be used as a panacea for all ills.

THE COMING-OUT BALL

1860 marks the debut of cocaine. This was the date that the Dama Blanca stepped onto the world stage, and the start of her intimate biography.

Early in that decade, Merck of Darmstadt began manufacturing a token amount of cocaine, about 50 grams per year, just enough to establish their marketing right. Today, the news of a new wonder-drug is relayed instantly to the world. But during the nineteenth century information dispersed slowly, and it took time for cocaine to become a pharmaceutical blockbuster.

During the 1870s, doctors around the world began exploring the potential uses of coca and cocaine – many failing to distinguish between leaf and powder. A Scottish physician called Robert Christison tested cocaine's effects on starving hikers and a Canadian doctor gave coca leaves to a lacrosse team prior to a game. Both concluded that cocaine and coca could be used as energy boosters. A French doctor saw cocaine as a cure for throat infections. A German physician surreptitiously slipped cocaine into Bavarian soldiers' drinking water, determining that the drug made them more alert and vigorous.

Articles on cocaine began appearing in medical publications in the 1870s. In 1874, Dr Alexander Bennett wrote a piece in the *British Medical Journal* identifying cocaine as a mild stimulant that could be poisonous in strong doses. Another article in the *British Medical Journal* examined coca leaves as a performance enhancer. This was put to the test in 1876 when American race-walker Edward Weston chomped on coca during a 115-mile, 24-hour race, to the fury of his British competitors, who accused him of having an unfair advantage. He has the dubious distinction of being the first man to introduce drugs to the Western sporting tradition.

PROFILE: ANGELO MARIANI (1838–1914)

Angelo Mariani was born in Corsica into a family of doctors and chemists and was apprenticed to the latter profession at an early age. There was little by way of entertainment in Corsica for the imaginative boy so he read a lot. From travellers' tales he learned of a plant, coca, that grew in South America and seemed to possess magical qualities. His interest in coca turned into an obsession.

Funded by his parents, Mariani moved to Paris, took rooms, and read all the information available on coca. With difficulty and at considerable expense, he obtained samples of the leaf picked at varying altitudes all over South America. He differentiated them by aroma – as with true experts in wine, he had an unusually sensitive nose.

Choosing the best examples of leaf, he steeped them in good claret. The wine leached the alkaloids from the leaves and, when filtered from the resulting sludge, disguised the inherent bitterness of coca. The clear appetising liquid contained very little cocaine, but cocaine and alcohol combine in the liver to form a potent compound: cocaethylene.

In 1863 he brought out Vin Mariani and knew he had a winner. It tasted like the finest wine but with an added kick that kept you sharp and provided a boost. The ingredients were entirely legal but only Mariani knew the secret process by which they were combined. Without protecting his wine by patenting it, he cornered the market due to his prescient use of advertising.

Mariani's marketing campaign was global in scale. He persuaded a couple of local doctors to sample it and give him his first quotes. He then despatched cases to a wide and eclectic range of well-known personalities. His accompanying letter on expensive stationery expressed his esteem and good will, suggesting that his Excellency might find a glass beneficial and bracing amidst his many duties, and requested a signed photograph for his humble admirer Mariani.

He had invented not only a unique product but the personalised celebrity endorsement. Almost everyone he wrote to replied enthusiastically, most likely while the wine's effects were still with them. The list includes Anatole Dumas, Jules Verne, Zola, Ibsen, the Lumière brothers, President McKinley, Ulysses S. Grant (it helped him finish his Civil War memoirs), Thomas Edison, Rodin and the Czar of Russia. Louis Blériot wrote that he'd nipped on the wine while first flying the Channel; Auguste Bartholdi, who had just completed building the Statue of Liberty, said had he known about the tonic 'it would have attained a height of several hundred metres'. And Pope Leo XIII was so uplifted by the product he sent its inventor a papal gold medal.

Vin Mariani proved an immediate international success and sold briskly not just in France and other European countries but in the US. Meanwhile, Mariani published the signed portrait endorsements in newspapers as fold-in supplements. He had them exquisitely presented and published in thirteen volumes. He gave one set to Queen Victoria, who was delighted to receive his books and said she valued them 'among the finest volumes in her collection'.

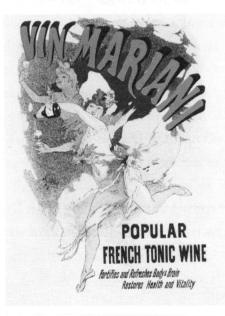

Mariani, the chemist/inventor and advertising pioneer, became a millionaire. Others were quick to follow and by the 1890s there were nineteen rival coca wines on the market. It became the staple fillip of the Belle Epoque.

TRANSPORTATION

Coca was an ace product, but shipping the leaves to the US and Europe was a nightmare. Consignments tended to rot to stinking compost en route. It would clearly be preferable to ship pure cocaine rather than coca leaves in bulk. In 1885, a chemist, Henry Hurd Rusby, visited Bolivia and, after first setting fire to his lab, formalised the method for doing so. Based on Niemann's process, Rusby created a transportable coca paste, known as *pasta básica* (basic paste) which is still smoked by the locals.

Rusby's coca paste put an end to the problem of shipping and by 1906 dozens of South American cocaine factories, particularly in Peru, were churning out crude cocaine. Germans chemists improved the process, doubling the strength of the product. The net result of this was that cocaine became cheap and readily available in the US and Europe. In Germany the price dropped to about 1 mark per gram. The stimulating product sold briskly but growing demand could not keep up with supply. There would soon be a glut of cocaine.

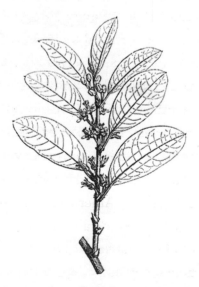

THE BOOM

By the late nineteenth century as many as 2,500 patent remedies, cures and tonics were on offer in America. The market for patent medicines was immense and virtually unregulated and it was in this environment that the new wonder-drug, cocaine, took off and flourished.

Cocaine was available over the counter, either in pure form or water-based solutions. It was welcomed as a treatment for asthma, alcoholism, the common cold, whooping cough, dysentery, haemorrhoids, neuralgia, seasickness, sore nipples, vaginismus, syphilis, as well as for morphine and opium addiction. It was also seen as a means to prevent female masturbation, since it numbed the clitoris. Herman Knapp, a German-American ophthalmologist who wrote a book called *Cocaine and its use in Opthalmic and General Surgery*, injected cocaine into his penis with predictably chilling results.

Two pharmaceutical companies, Merck of Germany and Parke-Davis in the US, cornered the cocaine market. Merck was particularly dominant and Germany would serve as the main global supplier of cocaine until the First World War. Parke-Davis used innovative marketing techniques, selling a bespoke kit with a syringe for self-injecting. They funded the *Therapeutic Gazette*, a medical journal devoted to extolling cocaine's benefits, and published a handbook on the drug, which was endorsed by the American Hay Fever Prevention Association. In the course of a single year the *New York Medical Journal* alone published twenty-seven articles on cocaine, all of them positive.

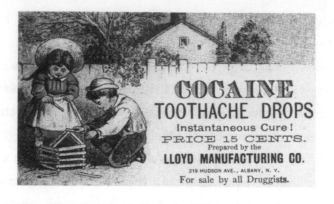

PROFILE: SIGMUND FREUD (1856–1939)

Even if a literal interpretation of Sigmund Freud's psychoanalytic theories is no longer applicable, there is no doubt that his ideas revolutionised the humanities and changed the way that we approach the human psyche. Most importantly for cultural modernism, Freud developed a theory of the fragmented rather than unitary self – comprising the superego, ego and id – and the subconscious. Turning his back on the Enlightenment's faith in reason and progress, he argued that civilisation is founded on desire – or at least the interplay between sexuality and repression – and that darker drives are always lurking beneath the surface.

Freud's reputation fluctuates between hagiography and demonisation, along with many caricatures in popular culture of the austere, bearded pundit in a three-piece suit and spectacles grasping a cigar while going on about sex. What often escapes note is the fact that, for twelve years (1884–96), and possibly longer, he was addicted to cocaine.

Freud's parents arrived in Vienna from the Ukraine as part of a great wave of Jewish emigration from Eastern Europe in the mid-nineteenth century to swell the ghettos of Western cities. Sigmund was the first of eight children and the family struggled to make money in an anti-Semitic environment. In these stringent circumstances, the introverted young man applied himself to study medicine, and was appointed to the General Hospital of Vienna when he was twenty-six.

In 1882 Freud met and quickly proposed to Martha Bernays, the daughter of a middle-class Jewish family living near Hamburg. Because he possessed neither fortune nor immediate prospects, her parents vetoed the match. For the next four years their relationship was epistolary rather than physical.

Freud longed for a financial fix so that he could afford to marry Martha and satisfy his natural impulses. Perhaps the largely unexamined new drug cocaine would be the answer to their problems. 'I am procuring some myself and will try it with cases of heart disease and also nervous exhaustion ... We do not need more than one such lucky hit for us to think of setting up house,' he wrote to Martha.

Freud's interest in cocaine was piqued in 1884 after poring over books on the coca plant and journals suggesting a variety of medical uses for cocaine – he was particularly struck by an article in the *Therapeutic Gazette* which posited that cocaine might be used as a cure for morphine addiction. Despite the expense, he bought some from Merck and used himself as laboratory rat. Once he felt sure that the results were favourable – it seemed to helped with his mood, indigestion and libido – he gave it to his nearest and dearest, including his sisters and Martha, in order to 'make her strong and give her cheeks some colour'. It was now time to try it on a real addict.

Dr Fleischl-Marxow was a handsome and brilliant young doctor until his career was cut short by an accident. While dissecting a cadaver, he nicked his thumb, which had to be amputated when the wound became infected. The continuing growth of nerve endings caused him to suffer from an unending torture of pain, which he treated with morphine. His self-administered dosage was high and he became addicted.

In May of 1884 Freud contacted Fleischl-Marxow and told his friend and fellow physician that cocaine was a possible cure for his morphine problem. Fleischl-Marxow clung to the news 'like a drowning man' and eagerly tried the new medicine. When Freud saw signs of improvement, he reported his findings in a lecture at the Psychiatric Society in Vienna, claiming that cocaine had improved Fleischl-Marxow's condition without causing habituation.

The contrary was so and by April 1885, Fleischl-Marxow was using over a gram per day, and combining the drug with morphine. Soon he was exhibiting classic symptoms of cocaine poisoning: fainting, insomnia and convulsions, combined with the conviction that insects and snakes were crawling beneath his skin. He spent hours trying to extract them with the point of a needle. Fleischl-Marxow remained dependent on both morphine and cocaine until his death in 1891.

Freud kept a photograph of his tragic friend next to his bed for the rest of his life – perhaps a sign that he felt some remorse about creating one of the first cocaine addicts. In the 1880s, however, he refused to admit to himself or the public that cocaine was anything but beneficial. In the summer of 1884 he wrote *Über Coca* (On Coca), a long paper on the history of cocaine which included the results of his self-administered tests and expounded upon his theory about cocaine as a cure for morphine addiction. *Über Coca* was Freud's first scientific publication and spurred him to write other cocaine-related articles, some of which are penned in a suspiciously frenzied style.

In the winter of 1884 and the spring of 1885 Freud felt positive about his research on cocaine, which had been reported in several reputable journals. His place in the annals of history seemed secure until a colleague, Dr Carl Keller, whom Freud had introduced to the drug, began conducting experiments with cocaine. He found it to be the ideal anaesthetic for operations on the human eye such as the removal of cataracts. Keller published a paper on the subject which gained him international recognition. Freud never quite overcame his resentment and blamed a long holiday with Martha for the fact that he hadn't made the discovery himself.

Martha was the recipient of many of Freud's

cocaine-induced mood swings and manic missives such as this from June 1884:

> Woe to you my little Princess, when I come. I will kiss you quite red and feed you till you are plump. And if you are forward you shall see who is the stronger, a gentle little girl who doesn't eat enough or a big wild man who has cocaine in his body.

In 1885 and 1886, Freud's cocaine use become more pronounced and his dosages increased. While working with the neurologist Charcot in Paris, he took cocaine to overcome his shyness and make social and professional situations more bearable. He wrote to Martha on the subject:

> He [Charcot] invited me to come to his house. You can imagine my apprehension ... and satisfaction. White tie and gloves, even a fresh shirt, a careful brushing of my last remaining hair, and so on. A little cocaine to untie my tongue ... As you see, I am not doing at all badly.

From 1887 Freud maintained an in-depth correspondence and close relationship with a younger surgeon, Wilhelm Fliess, a nose and throat specialist whose 'nasal reflex theory' hypothesised that the nose is a microcosm of the rest of the body and is, therefore, responsible for both mental and physical well-being. He wrote a book entitled *The Relationship Between the Nose and the Female Sex Organs*.

Freud naturally turned to Fliess when he had problems with his own nose. Excessive cocaine snorting caused blocking in his nasal passage and Fleiss would cauterise the affected areas with a hot metal instrument. Freud complained to Fliess about other symptoms, probably caused by cocaine, such as 'cardiac misery ... violent arrhythmia, constant tension, pressure, burning in the heart region, shooting pains down my left arm...' Fliess advised more cocaine and told him to give up cigars.

In 1895, Freud still believed that neurotic and psychosomatic symptoms could be alleviated with cocaine. He prescribed the drug to a troubled young woman, Emma Eckstein, who resultantly 'developed an extensive necrosis of the nasal mucous membrane' that needed to be treated. Fleiss was brought in to operate on her nose (as well as Freud's) and inserted a large wad of gauze up a nostril before applying cocaine to her wounds to stop the bleeding. It all went according to plan.

A month after the operation, Freud was called urgently to Eckstein's bedside. She was in dire distress because it turned out that Fleiss had accidentally left the gauze up her nose, causing an infection. Freud describes the moment of discovery: 'Before either of us had time to think, at least half a metre of gauze had been removed from the cavity. The next moment came a flow of blood. The patient turned white, her eyes bulged, and she had no pulse...' Fliess had botched the operation and nearly killed Emma in the process. The Emma Eckstein incident sickened Freud and haunted him for years to come.

Throughout the first half of the 1890s, Freud wrote alternately giddy and anxious letters about his cocaine use, sometimes claiming to feel unbelievably well, other times complaining of nasal swelling and the heavy discharge of yellow pus. He finally came to accept that the drug was both damaging and highly addictive 'if taken to excess'. He broke off his friendship with Fliess, another heavy user, and, in the autumn of 1896, wrote that 'the cocaine brush has been completely put aside'. There is, however, evidence that Freud continued taking coke for longer than he was willing to admit.

In later life, Freud was not proud of his relationship with the drug that had betrayed him. As if it were a love match with a deceptive woman, he never referred to that period of his life – indeed did his best to suppress any evidence of his misalliance.

PROFILE: WILLIAM HALSTED (1852–1922)

William Halsted was born in New York in 1852. His father ran a large insurance company. His mother – rich in her own right and somewhat grand – employed staff to raise the boy and packed him off to school as soon as possible.

The young Halsted was naturally brilliant but rebellious. He ran away from his first school at eleven and signally failed to apply himself at Andover. When he left at sixteen, his stern father kept him at home under the guidance of tutors who prepared him for Yale, where he was admitted in 1874.

There he distinguished himself on the playing field rather than in the classroom, captaining the baseball team and forming part of its gym squad and rowing crew. He was a fine athlete because of his quick and muscular build. He was also handsome, popular and gregarious.

Halsted was admitted to the College of Physicians and Surgeons at Yale medical school (his father was a trustee), where he chose to specialise in anatomy before studying in Vienna for two years. Freud was working at the Vienna General Hospital at the same time as Halsted but there is no evidence that the two met.

On returning to New York, Halsted established his own practice. He was well recommended by his wealthy clients and success came upon him almost at once. Furthermore, at this early stage in his career he made a medical breakthrough, discovering that human blood, once aerated, could be transfused into a patient through an artery – blood loss could be replenished.

In 1884 Halsted was thirty-two years old and at the top of his profession. In October of that year he bought some cocaine after reading about the drug and its success as a local anaesthetic. Like Freud, he was eager to obtain some and try its effects upon himself irrespective of cost. At this time he was working an intensive schedule, serving five hospitals as a surgeon as well as lecturing to his own students. While fulfilling this demanding agenda he embarked on a personal study of cocaine, mixing the drug with tap water and injecting it into a muscle and later a main vein.

Cocaine had an encouraging effect on Halsted and without difficulty he recruited many of his students into the programme to try it out. Very soon he and they were employing the drug on other occasions, either socially or to combat fatigue. The group formed a medical fraternity of users, many of whom progressed to addicts. There were several casualties and wrecked careers; a number of them died young.

A particular friend of Halsted's at this time was his senior physician, William Welch, who did not take cocaine. The bond linking the two men may or may not have been sexual, but Welch, then and later, behaved with nothing less than devotion toward his friend in his very rapid decline.

Halsted lost weight, muscle tone and colour. His normally cheerful demeanour turned morose. He became withdrawn and unsociable and behaved erratically. At Bellevue Hospital, after examining an emergency patient before surgery, he abruptly quit the ward and walked out of the building, only to go on a cocaine binge for several weeks.

Welch proposed a long sea voyage combined with gradual withdrawal from the drug. He would come along himself to control the daily dosage. The two embarked on a schooner and for a while all went well, but by the time they reached the Caribbean, Halsted was craving more. Wired and unable to rest, he chose a moment when all below were asleep, then stole into the skipper's cabin in order to break into the medicine chest.

By the time the boat returned to New York, the supply on board was exhausted and Halsted in a wretched state, trembling, agitated and paranoid. He was in no condition to return to work. Deeply concerned, Welch told him his career and life itself was doomed unless he agreed to enter an asylum for the insane and submit to a cure. He held out the promise of reward – if Halsted could get clean he could join him at the yet-to-open Johns Hopkins School of Medicine, where Welch had been appointed Dean.

Asking for time to consider, Halsted threw one last monumental cocaine binge then, pale and shaking, checked himself into Butler Hospital in Providence, Rhode Island, under the name of William Stewart.

At this point in time, insanity and addiction were regarded as largely incurable. Further, there was shame attached to addiction, seen as weakness of character. And there were no real treatments as such. But in his private room Halsted received care, attention and discussion with a sympathetic physician. He had a balanced diet and regular exercise, riding in the hospital's extensive grounds. He was prescribed chloral hydrate and bromides, though these failed to relieve his insomnia. He was tormented by restlessness and intense anxiety which informed every wakeful moment. To calm him, he was given shots of morphine. It countered the craving for cocaine but gave him a further addiction in that instant.

After six months Halsted signed himself out of Butler and joined Welch at Johns Hopkins, where he cohabited with his watchful sponsor in furnished rooms. In 1892 he was appointed surgeon-in-chief at the hospital and went on to distinguish himself as one of the greatest surgeons of his generation.

Halsted was credited with many firsts as a doctor. He was the first to perform a radical mastectomy and the first to insist on the use of latex gloves in a bid to improve antiseptic hygiene. He made doctors and nurses wear scrubs and caps and devised other aseptic strategies to keep microbes out of operating rooms. As a result, fewer patients became infected and fewer died. His stitching with fine wire or silk healed more quickly than with catgut and he treated human tissue with care rather than slashing through it recklessly like previous doctors had done. Halsted championed local anaesthetics and was an expert at wound healing.

Halsted's achievements did not make him happy or cure him of his drug-induced demons. He became withdrawn, suspicious, misanthropic and unable to look anyone in the eye. No charm remained, no trace of the extrovert and engaging man he had once been. He married one of his nurses but they inhabited different floors of their house. He lectured, but performed fewer operations himself. Some days he failed to come to work. He took long summer vacations in Europe by himself, staying incommunicado at different good hotels. At Johns Hopkins he followed an inflexible routine: he went home at exactly 4.30, and the rule decreed that *no one* might contact him until he appeared on duty next morning – or failed to show up.

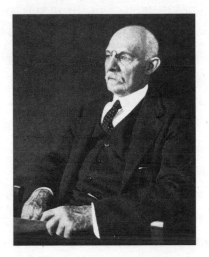

A heavy smoker, Halsted remained addicted to both morphine and cocaine until his death in 1922 at the age of seventy.

PROFILE: SHERLOCK HOLMES

That Sherlock Holmes was a coke fiend is a beguiling contemporary take on the popular old sleuth seated in his armchair wearing a dressing gown, discoursing on crime to ever-faithful Watson crouched at his feet. In reality Conan Doyle only wrote about Holmes's habit in any detail in *The Sign of the Four* (1890) and *A Scandal in Bohemia* (1891).

Holmes turns to cocaine during fallow periods in detecting because he hates being bored and needs 'mental exaltation'. In *The Sign of the Four*, his work is not going well and Watson disapprovingly notes that Holmes has been using cocaine about three or four times a day for months. He keeps his cocaine in a morocco case and theatrically injects the 7 per cent solution using a syringe. Watson does not look favourably upon cocaine and tells Holmes that it may damage his mind. 'Why should you, for a mere passing pleasure, risk the loss of those great powers with which you have been endowed?' Holmes, as usual, pays little heed to him.

Sir Arthur Conan Doyle trained as a physician in Edinburgh under Robert Christison, the same doctor who tested the effects of coca leaves on mountain hikers and wrote about his experiment in the *British Medical Journal*. In 1890, Doyle studied ophthalmology in Vienna, at the university where cocaine's use in eye surgery was pioneered. He ought, therefore, to have been familiar with cocaine's properties instead of referring to the 'drowsiness of the drug' as he does in *A Scandal in Bohemia* where he seems to mistake cocaine for opium. Doyle wrote in haste and did not always get his facts right. The error was remedied in later books when Watson speaks of cocaine as 'an artificial stimulus'.

Doyle may have originally chosen to give Holmes a drug vice in order to emphasise his Bohemian qualities. But as the century drew to a close and cocaine's reputation began to suffer, he probably thought it best to cure Holmes of his addiction and leave him to the task of solving mysteries. By 1904, Holmes has been weaned off his habit for good by Watson. Cocaine is never mentioned again even though Doyle continued writing about Holmes for another twenty years.

PROFILE: COCA-COLA

The original secret formula for Coca-Cola was devised by Dr John Pemberton, a confederate Civil War veteran with a morphine addiction and an interest in turning a profit. He marketed a product called 'French Wine Cola' which was almost identical to Vin Mariani, but had to change tactics when a prohibition law was passed in Fulton County, Georgia in 1886. Taking advantage of the soda fountain craze of the 1880s and '90s, he removed the alcohol and turned the drink into a syrup to be mixed with fizzy water, first selling his concoction at Jacob's Pharmacy in Atlanta.

Increase trade at your fountain by dispensing the delicious, refreshing beverage,

Coca-Cola

No fountain beverage ever increased in popularity so rapidly. None will draw so many customers to your fountain.

Advertising matter from any branch free.
THE COCA-COLA CO.,
Atlanta. Chicago. Dallas. Philadelphia. Los Angeles.

The active ingredients of his Coca-Cola were caffeine from kola nuts, and cocaine extracted from coca leaves harvested in Bolivia and Peru. Pemberton's recipe specified 5 ounces of leaves to a gallon of syrup, about

9 milligrams of cocaine in every glass. This is quite some hit. An ad for Coca-Cola ran in the *Atlanta Journal* shortly after, and claims for the new pick-me-up were striking: it cured indigestion, nervous exhaustion, headache, impotence and morphine addiction – a not uncommon affliction at the time.

Coca-Cola took some time to take off, so the impatient Pemberton sold the rights to a medical student drop-out, Asa Griggs Candler, for what seemed like the exorbitant price of $2,300. This proved to be a grave business blunder. When Candler died thirty-eight years later, Coca-Cola was worth $50 million and would come to represent American capitalism in the same way as McDonald's.

Coca-Cola was first sold in bottles in 1894 although the distinctive shape was not adopted until 1910. The expansion of the company was not without problems, due to the campaigning of Harvey Washington Wiley and the passage of the Pure Food and Drug Act of 1906 (see p. 30), which would force it to list the drink's ingredients. Because of the act, Coca-Cola switched from using fresh coca leaves to 'spent' leaves, from which the cocaine had been extracted. Only a trace remained but the taste for Coca-Cola had been established on the nation's palate and the brand was safe.

Another minor setback for Coca-Cola came when the company was sued for false advertising because the drink no longer contained cocaine. They achieved victory after a long legal battle and henceforth became fiercely secretive about their recipe and their operations. It is believed that they still use coca leaves for flavour and that Stepan Chemicals imports 175,000 kilograms each year before de-cocainising them. It is also thought that Coca-Cola was exempted from the narcotics legislation of 1930s in exchange for keeping narcotics commissioner Anslinger fully informed on coca dealing and cocaine production in South America.

The key to the Coca-Cola legend still lies in the secret formula devised by Dr Pemberton. It is said that only two executives in the corporation have access to the secret, each knowing only half the formula. A radio show, *This American Life*, in 2011 reported that the secret had been exposed by a newspaper in 1979, and that it matched with the recipe recorded in Pemberton's diary. Cocaine rumours, most likely unfounded, are still swirling.

BACKLASH

By 1900, attitudes towards cocaine were changing in the US. Negative side effects had been officially documented and there were a significant number of addicts, many of whom were doctors and dentists with daily access to the drug. More disturbingly to contemporary mores, their wives had also become addicted. In addition to some real cause for alarm about cocaine, the country was caught up in a wave of reforming zeal spurred on by the Prohibition Party. Before achieving their historic victory with the passage of the Volstead Act in 1919, they had taken up the sword against drugs, in particular opium, and the patent industry.

A broad coalition of people turned on the patent industry.

Women's temperance crusaders fought hard to prove that its claims were fraudulent and that dangerous ingredients were being slipped into supposedly benign products. Several journalists, including Edward Bok of *Ladies' Home Journal* and Samuel Hopkins Adams of *Collier's Weekly*, railed against the unethical nature of the industry.

The Pure Food and Drug Act was pushed through Congress by fiery anti-drug evangelist Harvey Washington Wiley and signed by President Theodore Roosevelt in 1906. The legislation obliged manufacturers to list the ingredients of their 'medicine' on the pack. The makers of coca wines, cordials and tonics went out of business in result, and a third of coca- and cocaine-based products were taken off the market. But in its intent to curb addiction the Act was a failure, for pure cocaine hydrochloride could still be purchased from a pharmacy. However, the Act set a marker: it signalled the end of an unregulated industry and, in the US government, the rise of the impulse to control and prohibit.

UNCLE SAM KNOWS BEST

The moralising zeal of American missionaries, coupled with the United States' desire to counter British influence in India and China, spurred the US government to organise a series of international drug conventions, the first in 1905–6, with the express purpose of ending the opium trade. President Theodore Roosevelt backed the Shanghai Opium Commission of 1909, composed of thirteen nations, which tried but failed to implement an international policy on opium.

President William Taft, who was so fat that he got stuck in the bathtub on Inauguration Day, could well have benefited from the appetite suppressant qualities of cocaine. Instead, he believed that it was the most dangerous drug in America and organised another drug conference at The Hague in 1912. Thirty-four participating countries with widely varying interests were merely asked 'to use their best efforts to control drug industries'. Understandably, signatories such as Germany were loath to say goodbye to a lucrative trade while non-members remained free to exploit the market as they wished.

The 1912 International Opium Convention revealed the difficulty of reaching shared resolutions on drugs, let alone enforcing them worldwide. The situation was not moving and it was clear the way forward must be set through national example, with America leading the way.

PROFILE: HAMILTON WRIGHT (1867–1917)

Dr Hamilton Wright, an inveterate boozer, was chosen by Taft to be his Opium Commissioner. The key force in setting up the Hague Conference of 1912, Wright also targeted the domestic consumption of cocaine, using fear of what it did to people, particularly black men, as his principal weapon. In 1910 he informed a congressional committee that 'cocaine is the direct incentive to the crime of rape by negroes of the South and other sections of the country'.

Wright's assertions obviously bore no relation to fact but the fabrication was so luridly conveyed by the media it touched a nerve of hysteria in whites. Racism was an easy emotion to evoke, especially in the South but also in the North now that black immigration to the area had increased. Cocaine had been given to black workers in New Orleans as well as to plantation workers in other parts of the South in order to extract more hours from them. Many had supposedly become addicted to the drug.

Wright had access to the scientific publications of distinguished physicians who said that cocaine altered the physiology of black men, increased their sexual voracity and lowered their threshold for pain. Hamilton Wright stoked the blaze with reports of the 'cocaine-crazed Negro' who lost all judgement when drugged, indiscriminately attacking and raping white women with feral abandon.

A favourite sensational claim was that cocaine gave black men superhuman strength and made it impossible to control them. Dr Edward Huntington Williams used the *New York Times* as a mouthpiece for his anti-cocaine tracts, writing that:

> bullets fired into the vital parts that would drop a sane man in his tracks fail to check the fiend ... Once the negro has formed the habit, he is irreclaimable. The only method to keep him from taking the drug is by imprisoning him. And that's merely palliative treatment, for he returns inevitably to the drug when released.

Such compounded scaremongering eased the passage of the Harrison Act, which he pushed through Congress in 1914 with little media coverage or even public awareness. The First World War had just broken out and people had other matters on their mind. But it was a seminal piece of legislation that marked the beginning of drug criminalisation in the US. And where the US acted, the world followed suit.

THE HARRISON ACT

The Harrison Narcotics Tax Act's declared purpose was not to ban cocaine (which was mistakenly classified as a narcotic), opium and other drugs, but to tax them. The legislation was a fiscal measure to include drugs as a source of government revenue, and its stated intention was 'to impose a special tax upon all persons who produce, import, manufacture, compound, deal in, dispense, sell, distribute, or give away opium or coca leaves, their salts, derivatives, or preparations, and for other purposes'.

The act stipulated that only doctors or licenced medical companies could register for the one-dollar-a-year tax, essentially banning everyone else from distributing drugs. Under the licensing system physicians could continue to prescribe drugs for medical purposes – i.e. cocaine could be used as an anaesthetic – but not to treat addiction. Because the act did not recognise addiction as a medical condition, addicts and recreational users were now placed outside the law and forced to seek their supply from the black market.

The act which had been intended as a progressive law to monitor a disorganised industry ended up putting addicts and the doctors who tried to treat them in prison. A Supreme

Court ruling in 1919 and a series of court cases came down on the side of enforcement, and by the twenties the nominal tax had morphed into a full-blown anti-drug law. Henceforth, drug use would be a criminal offence.

The 1920s saw the rapid growth of the criminal drug industry, a network of gangs engaged in organised crime catering to increasing numbers of drug users and addicts. Drug use spiked during Prohibition, probably because alcohol was so difficult to get hold of, and dropped after it was repealed. During the 1920s and 1930s, cocaine went underground, becoming the preserve of film stars (although the 1934 Hays Code banned overt depictions of sex and drug use in films), jazz musicians and members of the avant-garde. Elitist, glamorous and smart, a new culture emerged linked to showbiz and highlife, and further flavoured with an illicit thrill.

PROFILE: TALLULAH BANKHEAD (1902–68)

Tallulah Bankhead once famously declared, 'Cocaine's not addictive, darling. I should know, I've been taking it for years.'

Her mother died shortly after her birth in 1902 in Huntsville, Alabama. Her young father's reaction was to take to drink and women. Tallulah and her older sister Eugenia were raised by their grandparents. Her absent father lavished affection on Eugenia but ignored Tallulah, who overcompensated by misbehaving. She was thrown out of successive convents for exhibitionism, once for flinging an inkwell at the head-mistress and another time for flashing the gardener.

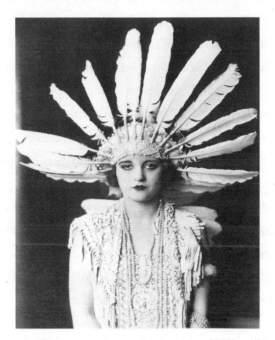

She was a chubby child but at fifteen lost weight drastically and transformed herself into a devilish scarlet-lipped seductress – a role she would maintain on stage and off throughout her life. Her grandfather financed her move to New York only after she refused to eat until he agreed. Her aunt accompanied her to reside in the Algonquin Hotel, on West 46th Street, the favoured watering hole of the theatrical and literary intelligentsia.

The environment might have been made for Tallulah, who soon caught the eye of Sam Goldwyn. He cast her in a movie. She was taken up by the 'kid flappers', who drank, smoked cigars and called each other 'darling' and said 'shit' and 'fuck' in conversation. Tallulah was sixteen years old but so sophisticated and assured that she came over as twenty-five. Invited to an audition, she set off in the same dress she'd worn for days. A friend who advised her to change was told, 'Who cares? He'll only be looking at my knickers.'

She was promiscuous though not an easy lay. 'I am the type who fattens on unrequited love, on the just-beyond-reach. The minute a man begins languishing over me, I stiffen and it's *finis*.' When attracted to a man she was bold in her pursuit, and equally unabashed in her affairs with women. 'My father always warned me about men, but he never said anything about women.'

Soon she was part of Manhattan's fast set, which included a young Noël Coward and the Earl of Amherst, who edited a social column in the *Morning World*. These were the pacesetters who emerged after the Great War to confound and shock their elders. They drank hard, used marijuana and cocaine, and many flaunted their bisexuality.

Tallulah was eighteen when the British impresario Charles B. Cochran offered her a part in a play by Gerald du Maurier that opened in London. She booked her passage on the *Majestic*, borrowed $1,000 from an elderly admirer and a mink coat from a girlfriend, and checked into the Ritz on arrival. Wild, flamboyant and outrageous, she embodied the spirit of the twenties and was welcomed into the ranks of the Bright Young Things.

During her ten years in London she appeared in seventeen plays, most of them clinkers, and gained some of the stage's worst reviews. For *Antony and Cleopatra*, 'Tallulah Bankhead barged down the Nile last night – and sank!' Of another, *Conchita*, she said, 'The boos would have rocked the walls of Jericho.' The critic James Agate condemned her as 'a joyless creature whose home is in the gutter'. Then in Michael Arlen's *The Green Hat* she achieved a huge success in a part which was a rendition of herself, 'I'm as pure as driven slush, darling.'

An offer from Paramount brought her back to the US, where she played in a total of nineteen films. She was a nightmare to employ. Her demands, drinking, drug use, fights and disgraceful antics provided frequent crises but she always delivered a performance.

In 1937 Tallulah was married to actor John Emery, whom she'd spotted from the stalls in *Busman's Honeymoon* to exclaim loudly, 'My Gawd, the man's divine.' Their marital bed was often shared with others; she enjoyed bisexual men and relished complexity. Once, at a party, an enraptured Groucho Marx gasped, 'I'd *really* like to fuck you!' Touched by his naivety, she assured him, 'And so you shall, you dear old-fashioned thing.'

In 1941 she separated from Emery, vowing not to touch liquor till the war was won, relying instead on cocaine and marijuana. After victory she resumed a bottle of bourbon *per diem*, while retaining her other habits and smoking a hundred cigarettes a day.

By 1960 she was suffering from emphysema but

continued to smoke, alternating puffs with oxygen from a portable cylinder. Two years later, wasted and frail, she stood on a platform next to her old friend President Jack Kennedy. As the band marched past, she indicated to the gorgeous young soldier playing the tuba and confided, 'Oh my, I wish he'd blow *me* like that.'

Indomitable, she made two more films, flying to Canada to recuperate between them. On arrival, asked by customs if she was Tallulah Bankhead, she replied, 'I'm what's left of her, darling,' adding, 'You don't have to bother searching my bags, there's nothing in them but liquor and drugs.'

In May 1968 she made her last public appearance on *The Tonight Show*. That winter she caught influenza and was admitted to St Luke's Hospital, dying of pneumonia on 12 December. Her last words were, 'Codeine, bourbon...'

BRITAIN

Until the middle of the First World War, cocaine could be legally purchased from pharmacies throughout England, as a medicine and dental anaesthetic. While the Americans had long been clamouring for a worldwide ban on drugs, the British did not want to harm the pharmaceutical industry and were not especially keen to participate in international drug conferences. They also believed that cocaine was relatively harmless, the tipple of aristocratic women and actresses.

PROFILE: EDITH YEOLAND (1873–1901) AND IDA YEOLAND (1876–1901)

The London stage has provided the setting to many shattered dreams. Struggling actresses Edith and Ida were undergoing a run of bad luck and had not worked for months. They shared a room in a theatrical boarding house in Bloomsbury, where they were behind with the rent and facing eviction. On 15 July 1901, the two attended an audition in London's West End for an American tour – and were not chosen. It was the final rejection after a litany of failures.

On the way back to their lodgings they legally procured three bottles of liquid cocaine from a local chemist. 'We are heartily sick of this weary struggle and our health is against us. Misery and misfortune seem to be our heritage and surely the best thing we can do is seek peace in nothingness,' Edith informed their mother in a suicide note. She blamed their unhappiness on 'something in themselves', claiming that they hadn't 'the nerves to push' any longer.

Mrs Callaghan, the proprietress of their boarding house, found the sisters midway through their descent into oblivion. The pair were brought up in consideration of others and had very good manners. Although gripped by convulsions and spewing pink froth, they politely suggested that she put them in a cab in order to save herself the trouble of disposing of their corpses. Mrs Callaghan demurred and instead called the police. Conveyed to hospital in a horse-drawn ambulance, nothing could be done to save them on arrival. They died the next day.

In life the pair had been confined to bit parts and understudy roles – the height of Edith's career had been a cameo in *Sweet Nell of Old Drury* at the Globe Theatre – but in death they gained an audience. Curious onlookers gathered on Great Russell Street as their flower-strewn coffins were removed in open carriages. This sad story served as a precautionary fable: vulnerable young women who move to London from the provinces in search of a glamorous career ... and the pitfalls that await them in the capital. Notably drugs. But it would take the First World War to bring drug use to the fore.

DORA

The Defence of the Realm Act, more commonly referred to as DORA, was passed by Parliament on 8 August 1914. Multifaceted and wide-reaching, its justification was the Great War and its declared purpose to aid mobilisation by clamping down on 'anything calculated to jeopardise the success of operations of any of His Majesty's forces or to assist the enemy'.

Only by citing a national emergency could the government get away with imposing draconian measures such as conscription, passport control, newspaper censorship, search and seizure and other regulatory practices, including strict licensing laws.

Prior to the war, pubs were open from the early hours until past midnight. Thanks to DORA, they were limited to two hours at lunch and three in the evening. The infamous 'Beauty Sleep Order' clause of 1915 stipulated that all clubs and restaurants shut down at 10:30 p.m. This emendation did not have the desired result and instead drove nightlife underground. Venues became smaller, more intimate, more specialised and more numerous. Many stayed open all night. That these clubs were illicit added to their appeal – by the end of 1915 there were over 150 in Soho alone.

On 28 July 1916, Sir Malcolm Delevingne, an anti-drug warrior who called cocaine 'the most baleful drug in whole of pharmacopoeia', pushed through an additional clause to DORA. Regulation 40b criminalised the possession of cocaine, opium and other drugs unless prescribed by a professional. Easily procured over-the-counter drugs now had to be bought on the black market. And the shipment of drugs such as morphine from family members to soldiers on the front, which had been a regular feature of the war, could no longer be effected with the same ease. Cocaine had become illegal in Britain as well as America.

VIVACIOUS, WANTON AND OVER-EXCITABLE

Cocaine featured prominently in the British press in the years immediately before and after the passage of DORA. The drug was demonised as alien and un-British, and responsibility for introducing it to the country was pinned on Canadian troops. A number of these soldiers based in Folkestone were busted in a juicily reported police sting involving a London prostitute who supplied them. The drug was hyped by gossip columnists such as Quex at the *Evening News,* who claimed that the 'exciting' and easily consumed stimulant could be found in 'discarded boxes in ladies' cloak-rooms all over the West End'.

Cocaine was believed to transform the character of its users and deflect their moral compass. Its male adherents were deviant 'pansies', degenerates, inferior men. The *Daily Mail* labelled cocaine use a 'vice of the neurotic, not a habit of the normal'. The *Daily Express* describes a typical nightclub scene: 'Round us danced the same old sickening crowd of undersized aliens, blue and yellow about the chin and greasy, the same predominating type of girl, young, thin, underdressed, perpetually seized with hysterical laugher, ogling and foolish.'

The nightclub was thought to be a centre of corruption and dissipation for young women, where they encountered men and drugs, and were transformed from wholesome, red-cheeked farm girls into wan, consumptive addicts. This was the case for Claire Plowman, the anti-heroine in Bloomsbury writer David Garnett's 1919 book *Dope Darling: A Story of Cocaine*, who becomes a cocaine user when she moves to the city and eventually corrupts her Scottish boyfriend with the cocaine that she keeps in a golden box hanging from her delicate, bird-like neck. The war breaks out and patriotism saves him from his vice – only after a grand finale involving a drug-fuelled sword dance and spattering blood.

Women were generally regarded as being especially susceptible to cocaine. Words such as vivacious, wanton, sensitive, over-excitable, hysterical were invariably used in describing females who succumbed to the drug. The most notorious cocaine 'victim' from this period was Billie Carleton, whose death provided Noël Coward with inspiration for his play *The Vortex* (1924).

PROFILE: BILLIE CARLETON (1896–1918)

Billie Carleton was christened Florence Stewart but chose her stage name because it sounded classy. She was born off Russell Square and was raised by her aunt after both of her parents died of alcoholism. She was given an adequate feminine education (she spoke French and German and played the piano) but turned to the theatre at the age of fifteen, where, despite an evident lack of talent and almost inaudible voice, she excelled thanks to her doll-like beauty and great personal charm.

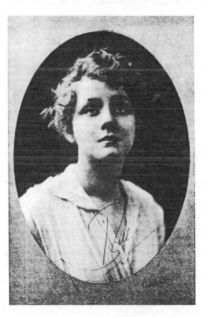

Charles B. Cochran, the same theatre impresario and showman who launched Tallulah Bankhead, plucked Billie out of the chorus and gave her the lead in *Watch*

Your Step, an overblown Irving Berlin production at the Empire in Leicester Square. She then went on to play in a Broadway farce and also starred in *Freedom of the Seas* at the Haymarket. She was now making the respectable sum of £25 a week and often featured in glossy magazines such as *Tatler*, on one occasion posing classically in a transparent dress.

By 1918, Billie Carleton's life was beginning to unravel. She had developed a reputation for bad behaviour, getting into spats with fellow actresses and gazing at Zeppelins instead of rehearsing. She was also deeply in debt thanks to expensive taste (living in the Savoy and going to Ascot in a Rolls-Royce) and a new heroin and cocaine habit picked up from her unsavoury friends.

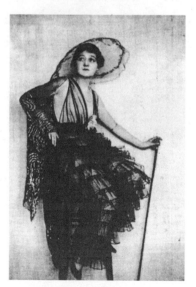

Like many childlike temptresses, Billie knew how to make use of older men. One mentor was John

Darlington Marsh, an ageing ladies' man who helped fund her immoderate lifestyle. Another, Frederick Stuart, a Knightsbridge physician who, while warning her against cocaine, gave her regular injections of morphine and liberal supplies of sleeping pills. The third character in this unholy triumvirate was Reginald De Veulle, a Jersey-born actor-turned-dressmaker of indiscriminate sexuality who had used his cocaine addiction to dodge the draft.

By the end of the Great War, Billie and Reginald De Veulle were at the centre of a gang of à la mode drug-takers, procuring their supplies from a Chinese man, Mr Lau Ping, and his Scottish wife, Ada, in Limehouse as well as from screen actor Lionel Belcher and his wife Olive Richardson. De Veulle used his own apartment on Dover Street to host drug parties which involved costumes, cocaine and opium.

The Armistice was cause for celebration for everyone across the country. Billie chose to attend the Royal Albert Hall's Victory ball in aid of the Nation's Fund for Nurses. Such detail was lost on Billie, who was too busy worrying whether they could get enough coke to make up for the lack of booze – the ball was dry. The day before the event, John Marsh came up trumps, paying £1,050 to redeem Billie's jewellery from the pawnbroker's.

The Albert Hall was decorated in blue and white. Revellers in fancy dress rubbed shoulders with uniformed guardsmen and military top brass as decadence and patriotism collided in pageantry and celebration. Billie's jewels sparkled brightly as she went tripping off to the men's lavatories accompanied by Reginald dressed as Harlequin. They snorted the finest cocaine out of gold boxes before joining Dr Stuart and the Belchers to watch the victory parade at midnight. The triumphant music of 'Pomp and Circumstance' and 'Rule Britannia' ushered in an assembly of allegorical figures representing Britain's Imperial might. Peace rode a shepherd-drawn chariot, followed by maidens with wheat sheaves, while others formed a living, undulating Union Jack triumphantly flagging the conquering home team.

Billie left at 3 a.m., taking the party back to her suite at the Savoy. There they breakfasted on bacon and eggs and topped up on drugs. She changed into a kimono and got into bed where she talked excitedly about her future on the Parisian stage or as a film star in America. When her guests left at 6 a.m., she was still awake and appeared content. Her maid heard her snoring at 11:30 a.m. and decided to check on her at 3:30 p.m. when the sound had stopped. When she couldn't wake her she called Dr Stuart, who gave Billie artificial respiration and injected her with brandy and strychnine. It was to no avail for Billie Carleton was dead.

AFTERMATH

Billie was found lying on one side with dilated pupils, blue fingernails, a stain at the corner of her mouth and a half-empty box of cocaine on her bedside table. The hotel manager said he had seen sachets of veronal (barbiturates) in her room the day before but they were nowhere in sight.

Billie Carleton's death was the first major drug scandal since the outlawing of drugs in the UK, providing shop window opportunity for the courts to prove that the new law was for real. In the following months, the Lau Pings, Lionel Belcher and Reginald De Veulle were all brought to trial on drug-related charges.

At first the press covered the story tactfully, suggesting that Billie had died from complications following influenza (this was time of the great flu pandemic). But at the trial of Ada Lau Ping, a host of sordid details about opium dens and pyjama parties emerged and helped feed the media frenzy about their 'circle of degenerates'. Mrs Lau Ping was described as 'the high priestess of unholy rites' by Frederick Meade, the prosecuting barrister who saw himself as a Victorian stalwart against an onslaught of depravity from abroad, calling the case 'disgraceful to modern civilisation'.

Reginald De Veulle was smeared in court and in the papers for his 'somewhat foreign appearance and accent' as well as for his 'effeminate face and mincing little smile'. Despite these aspersions, the jury was loath to hold the supplier responsible for what they were told had been an accidental cocaine overdose. Therefore they skirted around the manslaughter verdict by charging him with conspiracy. These were early days and penalties of the new drug laws were still being set by application.

The assumption that Billie died from cocaine – rather than barbiturates, as is undoubtedly the case based on the ease in which she died – misled the public into thinking that the drug was far more deadly than it is. The soft lens of history was more forgiving to Billie, who was transformed from a conniving hussy into an ethereal martyr. In the words of Charles B. Cochran, 'A more beautiful creature has never fluttered upon the stage. She seemed scarcely human, so fragile was she.' La Dama Blanca indeed.

PROFILE: FREDA KEMPTON (1901–22)

Freda Kempton was amongst the flock of young women from the provinces drawn to the London stage at the time of the Great War. She became a showgirl at Brett's, a famous basement dance hall. It had an all-female band, décor of pink and gold, and was all the rage when the Jazz Age reached London in the twenties.

Freda slept all day and worked all night. Like many of the girls she relied on coke. She adopted an exaggerated performing style and chewed on gum to disguise her constant jaw grinding. The coke had made her manic. Between her frenetic highs lay bleak despair. She relied upon a rich Chinese businessman and drug dealer known as 'Brilliant Chang' for financial support and cocaine. One day Freda asked him if it was possible to die from the drug; helpfully he told her only if ingested in water.

Freda spent her last evening disconsolately playing with her nephew before slipping away to take her fatal cocktail. At 9 p.m. she began screaming in pain, bashing her head against the wall and frothing at the mouth. She died in her landlady's arms. An incomplete suicide note reads: 'Mother, forgive me, I really meant no harm. The whole world was against me...' It breaks off mid-sentence.

Freda's passing was soon forgotten, but what remained vivid in the public mind was the image of the villain: the evil Chinaman who preyed on innocent young white women. There was insufficient evidence to prosecute Brilliant Chang yet he became a stock figure, not only in cartoons but in many thrillers of the between-the-wars period. In Freda's death another and this time male media stereotype was born.

THE OTHER

Edgar Manning (1889–1931) was the illegitimate son of freed Jamaican slaves, who came to London to play at Ciro's, a swanky nightclub. He gained a reputation for being a dapper, smooth-talking seducer. He had been a regular cocaine user and part-time dealer for years.

Manning was arrested when police raided his home and found drugs, scales and a silver walking stick filled with cocaine. The sentence of three years' hard labour didn't bode well for this skittish dandy with a weak constitution and refined tastes. He died in prison of toxaemia and heart failure in 1931.

By the time of his death, his reputation exceeded the meagre reality of the man. He was implicated (often retrospectively) by the press for nearly any cocaine scandal involving a white woman, including Freda Kempton to whom he sold only once or twice, and Billie Carleton with whom he had no connection. Edgar Manning personified 'the other' who could be used as a scapegoat for corrupting white women.

After the war, newspapers were rife with reports about white slave trafficking, Asiatic dope rings, spy scandals, miscegenation and rampant drug abuse. Stories about languorous Orientals in smoke-filled dens of iniquity, or sinister black seducers, helped propagate the idea that British morality was under threat from external forces.

The foreign and exotic was not entirely unpleasant and there was a degree of titillation to be had from stories of passed out, drug-fed women, dressed in silken robes suggestive of sexual misconduct. Filmmakers in both the UK and America seized upon the theme. D. W. Griffith's 1919 film *Broken Blossoms or The Yellow Man and the Girl* threw Lillian Gish into an opium den. *Cocaine* (1922), a supposedly anti-drug film, with a Chinese drug dealer played by a white man, was banned precisely because the censors thought that its scenes of drug-induced debauchery might give viewers ideas...

COKE AND THE JAZZ AGE

It is no coincidence that anti-drug fervour often takes place during tumultuous times. Cocaine-related media coverage was not reflective of a widespread drug epidemic, since its users were confined to the fringes of society and cocaine-related deaths few. Instead, it was representative of cultural anxiety.

The First World War brought the long nineteenth century to an abrupt end and ushered in a shocking modernity. The old order was gone, never to return, but what brave new world would rise out of its ashes? A dehumanising machine-driven dystopia à la Fritz Lang's *Metropolis* or the gleaming functionality of the Bauhaus, where rationality and mass production could be harnessed for the common good?

In the aftermath of the war, anything – whether frightening or glorious – seemed possible. The past had been erased and the future was a blank slate. The new woman with her bobbed hair and forward ways shimmied to the sultry jazz tunes that were flooding the airways and electrifying the night clubs. In the arts, the international avant-garde represented a strident assertion of modernity, innovation and experimentation.

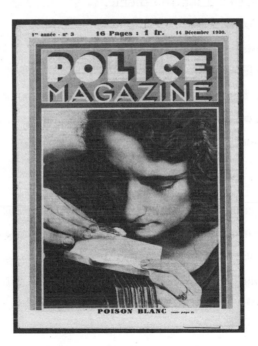

Cocaine is a drug that suited this fast-paced frenetic period in history because of its energising, tongue- and body-loosening effects. A hard-edged rather than a spiritual drug, it was taken by the hedonists of the Jazz Age, who knew that because God was dead, life needed to be lived in the moment. A taste for the exhilarated high induced by cocaine cut across continents. It was snorted in the metropolitan centres of New York, Hollywood, Paris and London, generally in 'artistic' circles, thus developing an association with louche recklessness.

The teens and twenties were the halcyon days of illegal cocaine, where even stories that ended badly (as most of them did) read as recherché and glamorous. Cocaine worked well with the cynicism of bohemian sets, for whom nothing was sacred other than decadence itself.

THE JAPANESE CONNECTION

From the 1860s, the majority of the world's coca leaves and semi-refined crude cocaine came from Peru. At the turn of the century other countries began growing coca in their imperial domains, such as British Ceylon and Dutch Java. By 1911, the Dutch were producing nearly a quarter of the world's cocaine.

Dutch domination of the Asian coca industry petered out due to international controls in the twenties. A demand still existed, both legal and not-so, and it was the Japanese who opportunistically stepped in to exploit this, planting coca in Iwo Jima, Okinawa and Taiwan. They made use of the double-strength Dutch coca leaf (developed from a Peruvian strand of the coca plant taken to Kew gardens) and by the late 1920s were producing roughly 1,500 tons a year, becoming a main source, along with Germany, of black-market cocaine in Europe and America.

The government and army encouraged an unregulated

drug industry and made it cheap and easy for the two major pharmaceutical companies, Hoshi and Sankyo, to sell their wares without bureaucratic hassle. Sankyo further benefited from licensing agreements with US companies Johnson & Johnson and Parke-Davis. Oversupply caused producers to dump their surplus in India, creating a cocaine problem where none had previously existed.

Japanese companies falsified exports records rather than comply with international controls set by the League of Nations, and in 1933 they quit the League altogether. Since drug abuse was not a problem in Japan, they saw no need to halt production. Distribution of the drug was a thriving covert industry that served two discrete purposes: cocaine sapped the moral fibre in weaker nations, and its profits funded armament and Japan's growing war machine.

WEIMAR GERMANY

During the late nineteenth and early twentieth centuries, Germany was one of the largest cocaine producers in the world because of its pharmaceutical giant, Merck. Unlike in the US where outraged moralisers railed against the drug, the Germans were relatively silent on the subject.

Germany's defeat in the First World War and the humiliating terms of the Versailles Treaty resulted in the creation of the democratic Weimar Republic in 1919. One of the stipulations of the Versailles Treaty had been that Germany comply with the Hague Conference's regulations on the drug trade, something the fragmented pharmaceutical industry was uninterested in doing.

In the early years of the Weimar Republic, Germany was

suffering from the after-effects of the war and the harsh reparations that led to inflation and economic collapse. The country teemed with war cripples, prostitutes and drug addicts – thanks to the black-market trade in illicit goods. Cocaine-related episodes in university hospitals rose from less than 2 per cent in 1913 to 10 per cent in 1921. By the late 1920s there were an estimated 10–20,000 coke users in Berlin alone.

A great deal of the cocaine bought by Americans and Europeans in the twenties and early thirties came from Germany, where domestic use was higher than in any other country. A number of future Nazi leaders, including Hitler and Goering who were young at this time, were heavy users/addicts of either amphetamines or cocaine during the Second World War.

PROFILE: ANITA BERBER (1899–1928)

It was coming up to midnight on a summer evening in 1922 in Weimar, Germany, when Anita Berber strode into a restaurant in the *Friedrichstadt* wearing a sable coat and high heels, with a baby chimpanzee clinging to her neck. She went directly to the bar, where she tipped the contents of her powdered compact onto its marble surface. She then arranged two lines and snorted them through a silver straw.

Moments later she discarded her fur coat, revealing her naked body. She reached for the nearest drink and one of the female guests dared to object. In reply, Anita tossed the contents of her glass into her face.

She gave the table an insolent sneer and sauntered off into the night with her chimp; she would look for her kicks elsewhere.

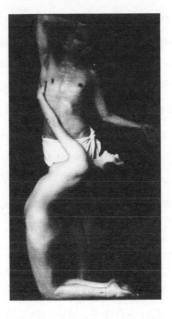

Anita was a beauty. 'She had a perfect body,' one admirer reminisced: 'Narrow snow-white shoulders, firm breasts with large, dark nipples, her buttocks were perfectly round, her thighs were beautifully arched, the shape of her legs faultless.' But despite her natural charms, she appeared intentionally sinister. Her signature look involved white foundation, green eye shadow and greasy red lipstick. Thomas Mann's eighteen-year-old son described her face as 'a bloody red creation conjured from a makeup case'.

Born a year before the new century, the underdeveloped, short-sighted redhead displayed an early fondness for mutilating dolls before finding her true calling as a macabre provocateur. At fifteen she became a star of Rita Sacchetto's under-age dance troupe, noted for its perverse eroticism.

Before the night of her opening, Berber decided to lose her virginity. She chose a plump, ageing novelist who provided her with flowers and adulation. Anita stepped out of her satin dress, slinked over to the bed and presented him with her porcelain body and spread legs. He was hooked.

In the early 1920s Anita became a Weimar celebrity. She graced the cover of countless women's magazines, received rave reviews for her performances and appeared in six feature films by Richard Oswald, a prolific and kinky Viennese director. Fritz Lang created a cameo role for her in his film *Dr Mabuse the Gambler*. He quickly came to regret his decision. Her drinking and drug habit made her wildly unreliable and – unforgivably in his eyes – she refused to shave her thick, blonde pubic hair.

Anita could be found strolling the streets of Berlin at all hours, sometimes wearing men's clothes and sporting a monocle, at others wearing nothing at all. She was catholic in her tastes for both sex and drugs. She consumed morphine, opium and absinthe, but cocaine and cognac were her true loves. Cocaine fuelled her stage routines, her craft and her addiction inextricably linked.

After a night of binging, Anita would retreat to her inner sanctum. Here she kept her menagerie of animals and an assortment of bric-a-brac: religious icons, totemic statues, burning candles, piles of fur coats and lingerie. According to the Czech choreographer Joe Jencik, the lucky few who crossed her threshold would find her in her boudoir: 'A wax-coloured white face without eyebrows or eyes, her body lay on her bed, or sometimes in the bathtub, with a whip in her hand, ostrich feathers on her head, a red corset on her back, cocaine on her tongue, morphine under her skin, passed out from cognac.'

Anita toyed with men and women alike, expressing a preference for the latter. She had affairs with Marlene Dietrich and other famous lesbians, but in 1920 ditched her female lover and manager for Sebastian Droste, a charlatan, poet and drug dealer. They planned an artistic magnum opus reflecting their mutual fantasies of sex, drugs, violence and death.

The Dances of Depravity, Horror and Ecstasy debuted in Vienna in November of 1922. Individual dances were titled 'Martyr', 'Suicide', 'Lunatic Asylum' and 'Byzantine Whip Dance'. In elaborate costumes (Anita once wore a nun's habit), they danced to the music of Rachmaninov and Tchaikovsky. Their two most applauded compositions, 'Morphine' and 'Cocaine', were especially authentic.

Life imitated art, and by the end of their collaboration both Anita and Droste were deeply addicted and in debt. Droste decided to seek his fame and fortune elsewhere. As a parting gift, he stole Anita's furs and jewels before boarding a luxury liner and reinventing himself as the tantric sex guru of a cult in upstate New York.

Without Droste, Anita descended into the mire of

addiction. Her behaviour became increasingly wild. She urinated on the tables, knocked over bar stools and smashed people with champagne bottles when she felt insulted.

Anita was aware of her addiction. 'You are a psycho-analyst. I know exactly what is wrong with me. I am thoroughly depraved. I snort cocaine. Look, one side of my nose is already destroyed!' Anita told a quack doctor that she no longer felt any desire and that her sensual performances were a sick masquerade. He told her to give up drugs. This was not an option.

In 1924, she fell in love with Henri Châtin-Hoffman, an American whose father had founded the German Evangelical Zion Church of Baltimore. Her dear friend Klapper, an abortionist known as 'The Stork', provided them with a honeymoon suite, where the couple gorged on drugs. They became dancing partners but were hounded by the vice squad, who prosecuted Anita for revealing 'her sexual parts and posterior' to the audience.

Times were changing and her persona becoming dated. Expressionism, with its exaggerated emphasis on gesture, no longer rang true with the post-inflationary mood. For three years Anita travelled the world, trying to revive her flagging career. While touring in the Middle East, she began coughing up blood and fell ill. She was dying of tuberculosis.

To the end she denied her impending death. Her gaunt face was smeared with lipstick as she lay on her bier surrounded by statuettes of the Virgin Mary and her collection of syringes. Weakened from years of cocaine, cognac and excess, the 29-year-old's ravaged body finally gave in on 10 November 1928 and she was buried in a pauper's grave on the outskirts of Berlin.

Dead but not forgotten, Anita Berber's sex- and death-laden performances had captured the Weimar spirit, embodying that very decadence that Hitler would stamp out, along with the black market drug industry, when he came to power in 1933.

2

WINTER SLEEP AND SPRING AWAKENING

THE BIG CHILL

After spiking during Prohibition, cocaine use in the US declined in the late 1920s, as it did in Europe. The Harrison Act proved effective and by 1928 most addicts were locked up. During the Great Depression, Americans were more worried about feeding themselves than snorting cocaine. Throughout the Second World War, patriotism trumped dissolute sniffing. Between 1912 and 1950, drug use in America was minimal.

Cocaine was restricted to a minority of musicians, showbiz personalities and rich partiers in the US. The 1930s through to the 1960s can be characterised as coke's years of oblivion, during which it dropped from public view. In 1957 Harry Anslinger, head of the Federal Bureau of Narcotics, went so far as to claim that the US had no cocaine problem.

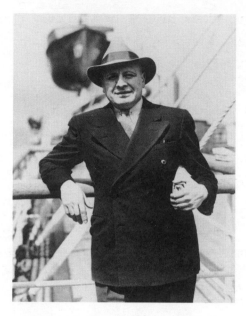

PROFILE: HARRY J. ANSLINGER (1892–1975)

Harry Jacob Anslinger was head of the Federal Bureau of Narcotics (FBN) for over thirty years (1930–62) and set the tone for the punitive and prohibitory stance towards drugs that is still in place today. Anslinger was a stern, authoritarian bully by nature and he made combating drugs his modus vivendi.

The FBN was mandated by President Herbert Hoover (1929–33) to enforce the Harrison Act. Anslinger relished his new role and set about building a bureaucratic empire devoted to the eradication of all drugs.

With the help of William Randolph Hearst he waged an inflammatory offensive against marijuana, using proven scare tactics. He claimed that 'reefers make darkies think they're as good as white men' and fabricated stories about marijuana turning meek young men into raging killers. In 1937 the Marijuana Tax Act was passed, effectively banning marijuana and hemp in the United States.

Successive Presidents Franklin Roosevelt (1933–45), Harry Truman (1945–53) and Dwight Eisenhower (1953–61) toed his line, making drug sentences increasingly harsh. The 1951 Boggs Act introduced mandatory minimum sentencing for drug offences, and later Anslinger imposed the death penalty for sale of the heroin to any person under eighteen.

America's political and economic dominance during the post-war years enabled Anslinger to strong-arm countries in recently liberated war zones, forcing them to impose drug control laws. Not in Latin America, however, which was unwilling to halt production of coca, a lucrative, long-standing and seemingly harmless part of their culture.

Anslinger's stewardship of the FBN coincided with a period of American confidence in its ability to police the world and spread the values of freedom and democracy. The way forward was the US way. America was God's own country, and America was clean. Heroin and morphine addicts were few, an unreported minority. Marijuana was the drug of blacks. This was the world as seen by Anslinger.

When Anslinger retired in 1962, cracks were beginning to show in the FBN's rigid, uncompromising edifice. In 1968, the Justice Department took over drug enforcement from the Treasury, turning the FBN into the Bureau of Narcotics and Dangerous Drugs (BNDD). In 1973, the BNDD was transformed into the Drug Enforcement Administration (DEA).

Anslinger's pet obsessions did not leave room for scientific research into the properties of drugs or the nature of addiction. Cocaine was entirely neglected except for its erroneous classification as a narcotic which led to misguided policies and a confused public perception about it in the future. The complacency of the FBN meant that America was ill prepared for the drug explosion of the 1960s.

CUBA LIBRE

Cocaine may have been hibernating but it was not entirely out of the picture. From the 1940s, Peruvian traffickers were supplying Cubans with cocaine and the drug became a staple in Havana clubs, which were thronged with inter-war mobsters, draft dodgers and rich lowlifes. From Cuba, coke made its way to Harlem, becoming the drug of choice amongst a select group of writers, artists and musicians.

During the 1950s, cocaine labs were multiplying in the jungles of Latin American, and supply networks solidifying. Cuba served as the main distribution hub during the drug-friendly regime of Fulgencio Batista, who assumed leadership of the island in 1952. A couple of prominent American gangsters, Bugsy Siegel and Meyer Lansky, were happy to escape the restrictions of their life in the Big Apple to relocate to a more benign climate of opportunity. With them came the Mafia, who introduced stability to the casinos and some security for visiting punters.

The Mafia ran the gambling and tourist trade with commendable efficiency, but the drugs trade was controlled by Cubans. The two respected each other's turf and both prospered until Castro seized power in 1959, when both were obliged to quit the island.

The Cubans took the drug trade with them to Miami, and expatriates would continue to control the industry until their business was hijacked by the Colombians in the 1970s.

FLOWER POWER

It was a cover article about Swinging London in *Time* magazine that first identified 'The Sixties' as a revolutionary decade utterly different from those preceding it. London, a drab dull metropolis, governed by a mentality born of austerity and the wartime virtues of going without, suddenly became another country – and it belonged to the young. Meanwhile, across the pond the transformation manifested itself in flower power and the hippy movement.

In 1967 the countercultural prophet Timothy Leary captured the zeitgeist when he urged 30,000 hippies at the Human Be-In in San Francisco to 'Turn on, tune in and drop out', an injunction that many took literally. By the end of the decade, the youth movement's sunny optimism was clouded by drug casualties. The deaths of Janis Joplin and Jimi Hendrix (to name but a couple) took the idealistic sheen off what had initially been regarded as a mind-expanding activity.

The sixties marked the beginning of America's love affair with drugs. Since then, drug use has scored a steep ascending curve across the graph. In the early sixties, about 4 million Americans had sampled an illegal drug; by the 2000s that number had shot up to 74 million.

In 1961, the United Nations (which had inherited the task from the League of Nations) finally passed the Single Convention on Narcotic Drugs, which set the terms for reducing the supply of illicit drugs through international cooperation. As a slight afterthought, Latin American countries were peremptorily told to phase out all coca production within the next twenty-five years. The Single Convention forms the backbone of today's system of international drug controls.

The Kennedy administration (1961–63) saw a relaxation in drug enforcement, particularly of marijuana, whose use was now widespread amongst the young. Lyndon B. Johnson's presidency (1963–69) continued this trend toward tolerance. As the sixties drew to a close, drugs were readily available in the streets and recognised as a reality of modern life. It seemed likely that drug laws would get more lenient and that in the not too distant future, most drugs would become legal.

THE COMEBACK KID

The drugs of the sixties were marijuana, LSD and amphetamines. Cocaine was neither generally available nor in demand. Musicians, their fans and partygoers of the period wanted a long-lasting high, which they found in speed. The Beat poets, major-league baseball players, long-distance truckers and Ayn Rand were partial to speed. Rand was hooked on Benzedrine for thirty years. In 1965 the FDA banned Benzedrine inhalers (as favoured by the abominable Le Chiffre in Ian Fleming's *Casino Royale*) and in 1971 amphetamine became a Class II drug under the Controlled Substances Act. Cocaine was a good replacement.

Some au fait scenesters, like folk singer Tom Rush, dabbled with coke in the early sixties. It was the title of his 1963 song with the lyrics 'Walked down 5th baby, turned down Main, looking for a place that sold cocaine...' The drug made its mainstream debut in 1969 in the opening scene of *Easy Rider*, when Peter Fonda and Dennis Hopper hide coke purchased in Mexico in the tanks of their motorcycles and begin their epic ride across America.

Soon the media began to pick up on coke's appeal, with publications such as *Rolling Stone, Newsweek* and the *New York Times* portraying it in a harmless and glamorous light. The 1972 blaxploitation film *Super Fly* starred a cocaine dealer and that same year saw the publication of *The Gourmet Cokebook: A Complete Guide to Cocaine*. Cocaine was still novel and relatively untested. And unlike heroin, it had lively rather than deathly associations. Heroin dealers were to be condemned – but the same was not so for the Snowman.

The majority of cocaine shipments came via human mules or amateur entrepreneurs who although in the game for profit were also drawn to the fun and risky lifestyle which accompanied the trade. The open market at the turn of the decade attracted a breed of young men – 90 per cent were men – who did not see themselves as criminals but as adventurers, piratical chancers challenging the rules of straight society. In a few years they were edged out by professional drug cartels in Colombia.

PROFILE: ZACHARY SWAN (1927–94)

Zachary Swan (a pseudonym used in the book *Snow Blind*), a mild-mannered, scruffy, blue-eyed chancer, came into cocaine smuggling relatively late in life – he moved his first load at the age forty-five. Riding on the carefree spirit of the sixties that lingered into the seventies, he discovered cocaine in its glory days but got out of the trade just as the mood was beginning to sour. His two-year career is representative of a brief window in the history of cocaine when dealing was up for grabs and amateurs could make a small fortune.

Swan's childhood was gilded but dysfunctional. He betrayed an early interest in betting, a habit which nearly got him expelled from Iona Prep in Westchester County. In his twenties and thirties he maintained a veneer of respectability by working for his father's packaging company. Meanwhile, he was hooked on amphetamines, gambling and beautiful women – he married one model in 1959 and another in 1960.

In the late sixties Swan settled down with Alice, a hippy chick in her early twenties who got him into dope and, by default, smuggling. Cocaine did not register in Swan's consciousness until he read an article on the subject in the *New York Times* by Customs Commissioner Myles Ambrose. Ambrose helpfully provided him and other would-be dealers with key information on how to acquire, cut and distribute the drug. He did some sums and was dazzled by the results.

Swan flew to Colombia on Avianca Airlines without even needing a passport and turned up on the beach in tie-dyed, cut-off shorts. There he encountered a disparate assortment of Western addicts, Haight-Ashbury homeless people, drop-outs and shysters. At first the cocaine novice was conned with bad batches but he quickly learnt to conduct purity tests, making sure the cocaine dissolved in cold water or bubbled and turned brown when burnt. He bought a gram scale so that he could work with metric units, the system of measurement that baffled most Americans but was vital for any coke dealer.

Swan's core business depended on the effectiveness of his first-class 'Mail Moves' from Colombia to the US which, in two years, were never intercepted. For his first he sent the coke in a box containing infants' toys and broken bottles of Johnson's baby powder. It would be too incautious to simply stuff the toys so instead he made corrugations in the box which he filled with coke. His packages were always delivered to carefully chosen 'front locations' such as the house of a college friend who ran a small cosmetics business.

Swan broke the cocaine down in his apartment, cutting it with dextrose or lactose, 6 grams to an ounce. He later switched to borax because it was easier to procure and mix despite the laborious preparation, which involved boiling, drying, pulverising and straining. He packaged the mixture in plastic sandwich bags and moved into a hotel where he distributed it to his dealers for $700–$800 an ounce.

He worked with a select group of reliable dealers and stayed away from the mayhem of the street. Some were friends with stable professions – one was a high-school teacher. Others, like Nice Mickey, were full-time criminals. Moses was a 6 ft 4 in. black man who socialised with Sylvester Stallone and Miles Davis and dealt in 'spoons'. Anthony, his most professional dealer, laundered his money, kept a gun in his pocket and bought pure, uncut cocaine from Swan in kilos.

In the autumn of 1971, a year after he had started smuggling, Swan was on a roll. He had been to Colombia six times and made multiple coke shipments without any trouble. Coke prices were soaring and a kilo was selling for $7,000 in Bogota and $30,000 in New York. Swan was making a healthy profit, but instead of opening multiple bank accounts or investing his money abroad, he meticulously inserted his cash into logs of wood. When the winter months approached, he grew anxious about his growing log stacks. Visitors were forbidden from making fires.

Swan attributed his success to smart transportation, particularly his ingenious use of wood. He employed Angel, who could fashion almost anything out of Madeira wood, to make hollow duplicates of standard objects such as rolling pins and statuettes, which could more easily be filled with cocaine than the originals. He used an old-fashioned flat-bed printer to compress the cocaine by 50 per cent and had Angel mail the objects from different locations to avoid suspicion.

Swan's druggie friends initially ridiculed his nerdy schemes but after a few legendary moves, they turned to him for advice about techniques. Black Dan copied his wood trick to insert cocaine into baseball bats for the California Olympic Games – no one noticed that baseball wasn't played in those Olympics. A friend dubbed Canadian Jack borrowed Swan's press to compress cocaine into Christmas cards, which read *May All Your Christmases Be White* and were signed by *Frosty the Snowman*.

Swan taught Canadian Jack about his 'Duplicate Bag Switch', a foolproof procedure designed to protect the carrier that is now a staple of the smuggling trade. Two identical bags (one has a scratch mark for identification purposes) are packed; one contains the carrier's normal clothes and the other is filled with the cocaine and clothes that are too big for the carrier. If the carrier is caught, she plays dumb and identifies her real bag on the conveyor belt.

The 'Brown Gold Coffee Move' was Swan's most inventive scam. He set up a fake office and placed a coffee jar on a grocery store shelf in Queens. An unsuspecting elderly couple bought the jar and found a brochure in it telling them that they had won a ten-day, gift-laden trip to Colombia. After a whirlwind tour with 'company representatives', the exhausted pair were plied with wooden knick-knacks, which they dutifully carried back with them to the States. While the couple were enjoying a celebratory lunch with Swan, his friend replaced the cocaine goods with identical duplicates.

In late 1971, Swan's luck began to turn. First, his good friend René Day was shot to death on a dark Miami street after leaving the Coconut Grove. Then Swan's hotel room was robbed and he lost $45,000 worth of cocaine. Finally, his girlfriend Alice was held at gunpoint and Swan narrowly escaped kidnap. The glamour was gone and the couple moved to Amagansett to get away from New York City. There Swan continued shifting cocaine but downsized his operation. He still managed a few more moves, such as the White Rabbit scheme, which earned him $75,000 and involved a single mother, her baby and a stuffed teddy bear. He also hosted coke parties in Amagansett for his dealers and close friends.

In September 1972, two years after his first smuggling trip, Swan and his friends were arrested for disorderly conduct on the beach, following a coke-fuelled night of revelry. The police refused him bail and broke into his house without a warrant. They discovered 500 grams of cocaine and a gun but failed to find the further 3 kilos in a wooden Madonna on the mantelpiece.

Swan faced fifteen years in prison. He managed to postpone his trial for over a year and made enough money selling drugs to employ a top lawyer. In June 1974, he charismatically defended himself by pointing out egregious police misconduct and finding some very reputable character witnesses. Swan was acquitted of all drugs charges but put on three years' probation for possession of a weapon. After his brush with the law, he decided to go straight. He married Alice and spent the next twenty years raising a family, tending organic vegetables and selling antiques. In 1994, he died from pancreatic cancer at the age of sixty-seven.

PROFILE: RICHARD NIXON (1913–94)

Would you buy a used car from this man?

Richard Milhous Nixon (President 1969–74) was not the most telegenic of politicians. Cartoonists depicted him with furrowed brow, mistrustful eyes, drooping jowls, elephant ears and, most memorably, a Pinocchio nose. 'Tricky Dicky' was also hirsute, remarking to Walter Cronkite before the first televised presidential debate in 1960 that 'I can shave within thirty seconds of going on and still have a beard, unless we put some powder on it'. Unfortunately, the application of a product called 'Lazy Shave' over his tenacious stubble gave him a deathly pallor – an embalmed look according to some commentators. Under the harsh lights of the television studio, he sweated so profusely that white beads of makeup started dribbling down his face. This televised disaster most likely cost Nixon the election to the less experienced but vastly more poised and attractive JFK.

Nixon did not take defeat lightly and came back in 1969 with a resounding victory, proving that looks aren't everything and that a man with a mission could win over America, especially an America polarised between squares and radicals. His stated cause was to support the 'silent majority' of hardworking Americans who hadn't demonstrated against the Vietnam War or participated in the destructive counterculture of the 1960s. He despised the Democrats as the party of 'acid, amnesty and abortion' and set himself to undo their liberal reforms such as welfare and the mollycoddling of criminals. Lyndon B. Johnson's Great Society needed to be dismantled. Now, poverty, racism, war were no longer to be blamed on society but instead blamed on individuals – individual addicts, individual criminals, individual law-breakers.

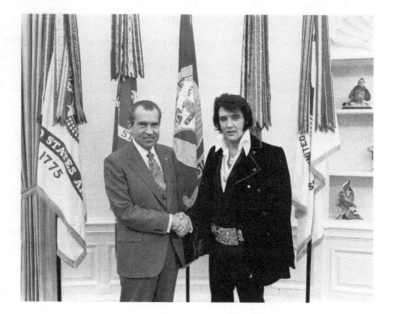

Richard Nixon with Elvis Presley

On 21 December 1970, the normally word-shy Elvis Presley personally delivered a letter to the White

House. In it, he expressed his anxiety about 'the drug culture, the hippy element and the Black Panthers' and asked if he could be made a federal agent. Nixon had found an unusual ally in the bloated and pill-addicted king of rock 'n' roll and arranged an awkward meeting where he was embraced by Elvis, who was wearing tight purple trousers, an unbuttoned silk shirt and a gold necklace.

On 17 July 1971, Nixon formalised his 'War on Drugs' at a press conference in which he requested funding for an $84 million initiative. He said drugs had 'assumed the dimensions of a national emergency' and labelled substance abuse as 'Public Enemy No. 1'.

On 1 July 1973, Richard Nixon merged existing drug enforcement agencies run by the BNDD, CIA and Customs into one super-agency called the Drug Enforcement Agency (DEA). The DEA was by now under the Justice Department, the law enforcement branch of the government, rather than the Treasury, a clear sign that henceforth the drug problem would be tackled with force.

PROFILE: THE LAUREL CANYON COKE COMMUNITY

'California Dreaming', the Mamas & the Papas' haunting and hypnotic 1965 hymn to the sunshine state, may have served as a siren call to the mostly out-of-state folk singers and rockers, including Joni Mitchell, David Crosby, Stephen Stills, Graham Nash and Linda

Ronstadt, who trickled into Los Angeles in the late sixties and settled in Laurel Canyon.

Laurel Canyon, which is located in the Hollywood Hills and overlooks the Pacific Ocean, was the perfect rustic retreat from the smoggy, traffic-ridden city below. Cheap wooden houses nestled amongst eucalyptus trees and blooming bougainvillea were transformed into communal party pads. Drugged-out hippies and Hollywood royalty such as Dennis Hopper and Jack Nicholson (who were busy writing *Easy Rider*) hung out in the hills and bonded over the new, pared-down music. 'I can only liken it to Vienna at the turn of the century, or Paris in the 1930s,' Graham Nash said.

Laurel Canyon felt like the wilderness but it was really a stone's throw away from the bars and coffee houses on the Sunset Strip, so people could go back and forth on their motorbikes – usually along windy, dangerous roads. The Troubadour Club on Santa Monica Boulevard became the stomping ground for would-be rock stars honing their craft and testing their country and western-influenced songs on the small but savvy audience.

Crosby, Stills & Nash, an early fixture at the Troubadour, released their first album in May of 1969 and helped define the new, lighter LA sound. Jimi Hendrix thought they were 'groovy' and described their style as 'western sky music, all delicate and ding-ding'.

Despite the laid-back vibe, with the rustic living and calculated cowboy aesthetic, everybody was trying to make it in a very competitive industry. Drugs, which had played such a role in the sixties, were shifting from hallucinogens and pot to pot and a new drug called cocaine. This mysterious substance was far too expensive for laymen and, for the time being, remained the preserve of rock stars and movie stars. Luckily, Laurel Canyon boasted its fair share of both. Crosby and Stills were such admirable sniffers that, by 1969, they had been dubbed 'the Frozen Noses'.

Laurel Canyon and the further afield Topanga Canyon were inhabited by an assortment of musicians, actors and LSD-damaged oddballs. Everybody with long hair and a groovy outlook was accepted, which sometimes made it difficult to distinguish between the truly cool and the truly deranged. People became less trusting of each other after Charles Manson, a charismatic ex-convict who had wheedled his way into the scene through Dennis Wilson of the Beach Boys and Neil Young, brutally murdered Roman Polanski's pregnant wife and her four friends on 9 August 1969.

The Manson murders, along with the disaster of Altamont, where the Rolling Stones hired warring factions of the Hell's Angels motorbike gang to police their concert, brought the sixties experiment to a close. The carefree days were over and it was time to be a little more guarded and calculating, even when it came to making music. There was nothing more calculating than the formation of the Eagles, a group that, from the very beginning, was designed to succeed. 'We wanted it all. Peer respect. AM and FM success, No. 1 singles and albums, great music and a lot of money. Why not try for the top?' lead singer Glenn Frey explained.

Other bands had fused country and rock but the Eagles got the formula for mainstream success right. Their tunes were catchy and their lyrics were simultaneously generic and edgy, conjuring up images of a mythic but slightly sinister California where, if you weren't careful, you might end up 'on a dark desert highway' en route to a hotel you could never leave. One of the Eagles' first hit songs, 'Witchy Woman' (1972), had several not very subtle references to cocaine, including 'see how high she flies' and 'she drove herself to madness with a silver spoon'.

Drugs were a fact of life in Laurel Canyon and some musicians seemed hell-bent on self-destruction. Gram Parsons, a troubled southerner with a trust fund who posthumously became a country-rock hero, was usually high on a combination of cocaine, magic mushrooms and heroin. His friend-worship of coke fiend Keith Richards only furthered his addiction.

In September of 1973, Parsons met his end at a motel in Joshua Tree National Park, a beautiful desert outside of LA, after injecting a speedball of heroin and cocaine. Two female companions tried to revive him by shoving ice cubes up his anus when they noticed that he had turned blue. It didn't work and the 26-year-old was shortly pronounced dead. His body was snuck out of the morgue and set alight in his beloved Joshua Tree as per Parsons's prescient request.

Gram Parsons was an early cocaine casualty but many in the extended circle were becoming, in the words of Linda Ronstadt, 'deaf, dumb and real obnox-ious' because of too much cocaine. Linda had to have her nose cauterised twice while supporting Neil Young on his 1973 tour. Even Joni Mitchell, who was mostly shielded from drug use by her protective boyfriends, dabbled in cocaine. 'I wrote some songs on cocaine because initially it can be a creative catalyst,' she said. 'In the end it'll fry you, kill the heart. It kills the soul and gives delusions of grandeur as it shuts down your emotional centre. Perfect drug for a hitman but not so good for a musician,' she said.

By 1973, cocaine had infiltrated the musical community at large. Mo Ostin at Warner-Reprise Records was fed up with the endless sniffing during work hours and David Geffen, founder of Asylum Records, said that 'there was a period when people would proudly wear their little gold spoons around their neck'. Geffen's business partner, Elliot Roberts, confirmed that cocaine use was everywhere. 'For a while no one could say a bad thing about it. No one realised that it was totally addictive ... Everyone was like, "Wanna bump?" It was so mainstream.'

Vials of coke were passed around like candy at clubs and the drug became a stand-in for glamour and an aid to sexual conquest. The Roxy club, which had an exclusive VIP area called On the Rox, opened on the Sunset Boulevard in 1973 and became the 'it' spot for the cocaine glitterati. Partly owned by David Geffen, the Roxy was a place for posturing and snorting rather than discovering musical talent. To many, it represented everything that was wrong with a musical scene that had been corrupted by money and drugs.

Neil Young, who joined Crosby, Stills & Nash in 1969, said that the band was ruined by cocaine and egos. When they went on what would turn out to be their final tour, known as the 'Doom Tour', in 1974, they took so much coke that Joni Mitchell, their support act, said that they had nosebleeds on stage. Crosby, who had snorted continuously since 1966, had to stop snorting in 1976 when he perforated his septum. He solved this problem by ingesting it in its liquid form and then becoming an avid freebaser, smoking an ounce a day for many years.

The Eagles matched Crosby, Stills, Nash & Young in cocaine consumption. With the release of 'One of Those Nights' in 1975 and 'Hotel California' in 1976, they were the biggest group in America. The band members, although still in their late twenties, were now millionaires. They lived in a mansion in Bel Air, were serviced by gorgeous chicks and snorted mountains of cocaine. 'Those were the horniest boys in town, living life without rules or limits', according to one ex-girlfriend.

Eagles drummer Don Henley was a notorious womaniser. He had an affair with Stevie Nicks just as Fleetwood Mac was beginning to give the Eagles some competition. This period was, according to Glenn Frey, the apogee of rock 'n' roll excess, a period where 'wine was the best, drugs were good, the women were beautiful and, man, we seemed to have an endless amount of energy'. Their 'energy' came from liberal supplies of coke.

The commercial triumph of the Eagles did not prevent critics from deriding them as soulless, predictable sell-outs. Their music seemed to mark the end of the intimate singer-songwriter genre and the beginning of mass-market, corporate rock for large arenas, fawning crowds and big bucks. It didn't help that Frey and Henley were behaving like amoral, coke-addled bastards who, of course, could no longer stand the sight of each other. On 21 November 1979, as the band skidded towards dissolution, Henley was arrested after a naked sixteen-year-old girl, high on cocaine and Quaaludes, was found at his home.

Disillusionment had set in amongst the Laurel Canyon musicians and they sang of ennui, death and cocaine. In 1977 Jackson Browne came out with an album titled *Running on Empty*. In one song, 'Cocaine', he can be heard sniffing a line. Lowell George of the band Little Feat had been using more and more cocaine and died of a heart attack on 29 June 1979. He was thirty-four years old. And on 23 November, Judee Sill, a folk singer with a religious bent, died of codeine and cocaine intoxication in her North Hollywood apartment.

Cocaine didn't directly destroy the innocence of the Laurel Canyon music scene, but it didn't help. The drug, more than anything else, reflected the cynicism and numbness that had entered their systems and, by the mid-seventies, killed off their idealism.

PROFILE: STEVIE NICKS (1948—)

The young Stevie Nicks was pretty as a doll with her big kohl-lined eyes, a wide snub nose, a babyish pout and a mass of feathery blonde hair. She was part all-American cheerleader pixie, part 1960s love child, part gypsy witch and 100 per cent rock goddess – a perfect sex object to her legions of male admirers.

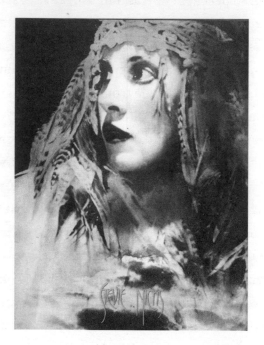

Stevie usually wore pointed six-inch suede platform boots (she was only 5 ft 1 in. after all) and billowing chiffon dresses designed by Margaret Kent. She had a penchant for lace, wide felt hats, sleeves that looked like bat's wings, capes, paisley prints, dark satin robes with hoods and anything mystical, gothic or fairy-like.

Stevie may have seemed delicate and dreamy but her little body housed an almighty voice, a voice that was raspy, melodic and full of passion. She was also a very gifted songwriter. When she performed her signature song, 'Rhiannon' – supposedly about a Welsh witch – her bandmates said she seemed possessed. With flying arms, flying locks and flying garments, she would spin around to the throbbing guitar riffs like she was in a trance. And perhaps she was. But she also saw herself as an old-school entertainer whose duty it was to give her audience a proper show. If she hadn't been a rock star, she thought she might have ended up on Broadway, or, in a past life, in a vaudeville troupe.

As a child, Stephanie (Stevie) Lynn's twin passions were singing – she loved Janis Joplin – and dressing-up. Her upbringing was comfortable: her mother kept house and her businessman father was Vice-President of Greyhound Buses. In high school Stevie met hand-some guitar virtuoso Lindsey Buckingham and the fated duo moved to LA as lovers and bandmates.

Fleetwood Mac was a British blues band that had already had several incarnations since its formation in the 1960s. Now that Mick Fleetwood and Christine and John McVie had relocated to LA, they needed a new sound and a new guitar player. Buckingham fit the bill perfectly and Stevie was part of the package.

Fleetwood Mac's classic, record-smashing album *Rumours* (1977) sold more records than any other album until Michael Jackson's *Thriller*, and catapulted them into superstardom. The album, which famously documents their torturous, unravelling personal lives – Christine and John as well as Stevie and Lindsey were breaking up – was also written under the influence of an inordinate amount of cocaine.

During recording sessions, their studio engineer, who kept the band's coke in a velvet bag under the sound equipment table, was responsible for keeping them regularly 'refreshed'. Because coke had been so instrumental to the album's tone, they wanted to give their dealer credit in the liner notes, a request their producer refused to grant. The dealer died in a gang execution before the album came out.

With eleven near-perfect tracks, including 'The Chain', 'Second Hand News', 'You Make Loving Fun' and 'Never Going Back', *Rumours* fused British pathos with American energy, creating a ragingly popular sound that would have veered on cheesy if it hadn't been so rooted in traditional rock 'n' roll and blues. One of Stevie's songs, 'Gold Dust Woman,' started out with the lines 'Rock-on, gold dust woman, Take your silver spoon and Dig your grave', a direct reference to cocaine. These dire words could be taken as a sign of self-awareness about the dangers of the drug but, as it turned out, that came much later. For the time being, Stevie, like many other users, was convinced that cocaine was recreational and non-addictive. She was caught up in the good times.

Fleetwood Mac had a heavy touring schedule and the band members used cocaine to keep themselves going. Their manager, who was worried about overconsumption, limited them to a few lines of coke before each show. Somehow, they always managed to get more. During the 1979 'Tusk' tour, with fame and endless adulation going to her head, Stevie demanded that all of her hotel suites be painted pink and fitted with white, baby grand pianos. The world-famous band was living in the lap of luxury, ordering plates of gourmet food that nobody ate and practically swimming in champagne and cocaine.

From 1980 onwards, Stevie was hopelessly addicted to coke. 'It was like being swept up on a white horse by a prince. There was no way to get off the white horse – and I didn't want to. It took over my life in a big way,' she later remarked. Fortunately, Stevie and the band were rolling in money. She estimates that she spent at least a million, perhaps much more, on cocaine. Mick Fleetwood, who earned less money than Stevie because he didn't write any songs, spent about $8 million on coke and went bankrupt twice because of it.

The mid-eighties was a time of reckoning for Stevie. She had been addicted to cocaine for ten years and had gotten to the point where 'all you can do is think about where your next line is coming from'. It was also ruining the lives of those around her – John McVie had a substance-related seizure and was arrested in Hawaii for the possession of 4.5 grams of cocaine and illegal weapons. Her real moment of truth came in 1986 when a plastic surgeon told her that unless she gave up cocaine, her nose would fall off her face – she still has a hole in her septum the size of a ten-pence coin.

Stevie Nicks checked herself into the Betty Ford Center in Palm Springs, finding herself alongside James Taylor's backing singers and Tammy Wynette. After thirty days in this anti-substance boot camp, she came out clean and never touched cocaine again.

Unfortunately, she switched one addiction for another, spending nearly ten more years hooked on Klonopin, a tranquilliser prescribed to her by her psychiatrist.

Now in her mid-sixties, Stevie Nicks feels lucky to be alive after everything she put her body through. But does she regret having used so much coke? No, she does not. It was part of making music, part of being a rock star and perhaps even made her who she is. 'I wouldn't go back and change anything,' she said in 1997. She still denies the persistent but uncorroborated rumour that in her heyday she had to pay an assistant to shoot cocaine up her ass after other methods had ceased to be effective.

GERALD FORD (1913–2006) AND JIMMY CARTER (1924–)

The resignation of Nixon in 1974 led to a lull in the War on Drugs as more liberal policies were adopted by his successor Gerald Ford (President 1974–77), who was portrayed by the press as a bumbling simpleton from Omaha. During his short presidency, which never quite recovered from his public pardoning of Richard Nixon, his administration published its White Paper on Drug Abuse (1976), which argued that marijuana and cocaine are relatively harmless. The paper stated that cocaine is not physically addictive and that it 'usually does not result in serious social consequences'.

Now that shipments from Latin America were increasing, so was the drug's popularity and media coverage. In May

1977 *Newsweek* ran a cover story, reporting, 'a little cocaine is now de rigueur at some LA dinner parties,' comparing it to Dom Pérignon champagne because of its classy associations. All of this free advertising worked and cocaine use amongst the young doubled between 1977 and '79.

Jimmy Carter's well-intentioned efforts towards a rational approach to the War on Drugs during his presidency of 1977–81 began with a bid to legalise marijuana. This did not happen. He didn't even manage to halt Operation Condor, an unpopular drug spraying operation that started in 1975 and continued well into the eighties. It devastated Mexican poppy and marijuana fields, which led to a spike in the price of pot in America and encouraged users to switch to cocaine.

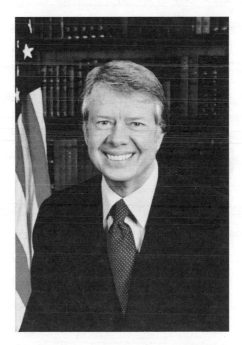

Jimmy Carter

PROFILE: PETER BOURNE (1939–)

Peter Bourne was a gentle, self-deprecating Oxford-educated Brit who had gone to medical school in Georgia, where he became a key figure in the Democratic Party, working for then Governor Jimmy Carter and helping in his bid for the presidency. Carter rewarded him by making him White House Health Policy Adviser on drugs, a position that he was well qualified to fill, having run successful drug treatment programmes in Georgia.

Like many in Carter's administration, Bourne saw nothing wrong with recreational drug use, at one point remarking that 'cocaine is probably the most benign of the illicit drugs' and implying that it should be legalised. He was an excellent physician and a committed liberal but not particularly savvy when it came to the cut-throat world of politics. He had already got into trouble for using a false name to prescribe sedatives to a White House acquaintance when he accepted an invitation that would get him into deeper hot water.

NORML, the National Organisation for the Reform of Marijuana Laws, was a radical pressure group started in 1971 by the charismatic Keith Stroup with a $5,000 donation from the Playboy Foundation. In the space of a few years it had become a powerful lobby that wielded great influence in the Carter administration and seemed on the brink of pushing through the legalisation of marijuana. In 1977, NORML successfully straddled the Establishment and the counterculture. Their annual Christmas party was Washington's event of the season and was bound to be a drug-fuelled bash.

Over 400 guests, including politicians, lawyers, journalists, yuppies, political activists, drug smugglers and celebrities, had been invited to a large, gutted townhouse on the freezing December night. They were greeted by waiters carrying silver trays with caviar and hand-rolled joints made from the finest Laos-grown marijuana – a special gift from an avid NORML supporter who was a Vietnam vet turned pot farmer in the Deep South. Because everyone at the party was affiliated with drugs in some way, either politically or socially, there was a wide selection on hand including pot, hallucinogens and cocaine.

High and inebriated guests shared drugs with each other while dancing under the strobe lights to a live rock band. The party was a resounding success and long-haired 34-year-old Keith Stroup, who was wearing jeans, a blue velvet jacket and a red bow tie, was in his element, flirting with Hugh Hefner's foxy and business-minded daughter Christie, and bantering with Gonzo journalist Hunter S. Thompson. When his colleague told him that Peter Bourne had arrived and was look ing for some cocaine, he asked his friend Tom Forcade, a journalist for *High Times* magazine, if he had any. Forcade, a gaudy figure in a white hat and snakeskin boots, had unfortunately run out. Stroup couldn't leave such a star guest wanting so he contacted a dealer to ask for 8 grams of the finest.

When the coke arrived, Stroup suggested to Bourne and their small posse that they go somewhere more private. They ascended a staircase in full view of the entire party, which included the editor of the *Washington Post*. Upstairs, Hunter S. Thompson got engrossed in a football game and the others made small talk. Then Stroup's contact brought out a cocaine 'bullet' that, when twisted, spat out a calibrated dose of white powder. They passed the bullet round the group 'til it reached Bourne. Everyone's attention was on the President's drug czar – would he really take a hit in front of them? For a moment Bourne paused, perhaps considering the implications of his action, before accepting the offering and partaking. The group relaxed and continued to take more using a mirror and then a coke spoon. When all were all good and high, they made their equally public descent down the open staircase to rejoin the party.

Gossip about the incident started almost immediately but it took some months for the story to break. It might have been kept under wraps – due to a lack of proof – if Stroup hadn't decided to take revenge on Bourne for continuing to support marijuana spraying in Mexico. Questioned by a reporter, Stroup confirmed the event and the story broke in the *Washington Post*.

The Bourne scandal shook the Carter administration to its core, confirming conservative suspicions that he was sanctioning drug abuse. Both Bourne and Stroup lost their jobs and Carter was forced to do an about-face on his liberal drug programmes. Never again would American politicians try to be cool.

PROFILE: HAMILTON JORDAN (1944–2008)

President Carter didn't have much luck with his advisers, who mostly came from his home state of Georgia and were trying to do away with the stuffy pomp and ceremony of Washington by acting consciously down-to-earth and normal. Hamilton Jordan was a wunderkind who had run Carter's gubernatorial campaign at the age of twenty-six and became President Carter's Chief of Staff in his thirties.

Jordan influenced Carter's policy decisions but was also a bit of liability. The White House had to issue a paper refuting the accusation that he had spat out his drink into a woman's face. And it was widely reported that he had offended the ambassador to Egypt's wife by gazing at her ample bosom and saying, 'I have always wanted to see the pyramids.'

A more damaging rumour circulated by the media was that Jordan had taken cocaine and had casual sex at Studio 54 during a 1978 visit to the club. A long and expensive investigation in 1979 failed to find evidence to support this and the charges were dropped. But the damage was already done and Carter was embarrassed once again.

PROFILE: STUDIO 54

Any New Yorker over the age of fifty will have bored you with tales about New York in the seventies. They will tell you that city was rough, dangerous, down and out, crime infested, sick. Addicts roamed the streets of Soho and anyone who had their wits about them would stay clear of the area past dusk, unless they were looking for a fix. Public services were broken and the streets were mean, but out of the ashes emerged the coolest art and music scene that has ever existed.

A conversation with an old New Yorker may go something along the lines of...

You grew up surrounded by Starbucks and poodles while we dodged knife-wielding maniacs. Who is Rihanna when we had Debbie Harry? Did you shoot heroin with Lou Reed at a loft party in the East Village? Did you hear the Talking Heads perform at the Ocean Club in Tribeca in 1977 and the Ramones at CBGB? Did you participate in Gordon Matta-Clark's 1974 'deconstruction' when he cut off the front of a condemned house? Did you have a brief affair with Laurie Anderson? Did you snort coke at Studio 54 with Edie Sedgwick and end up compromised in the rubber lounge with dragstar Queen of Sheba? I didn't think so.

Studio 54 was an epoch-defining club that dominated New York nightlife for three glorious years between 1977 and 1980. It encapsulated a brief but very charged era when pleasure was up for grabs, in part because sex and cocaine seemed like risk-free pursuits. The club was a space where gender and race were discarded, where the transgressive was the norm and where celebrities mingled with the riff-raff – so long as they were fabulous.

Steve Rubell and Ian Schrager were the men behind the magic. They were both Jewish boys from Brooklyn who had met at Syracuse University in the late sixties. Rubell was gay and charismatic, Schrager was straight and serious and together they made an ideal business partnership. They set up a couple of clubs in Boston and Queens but knew they needed to crack Manhattan for the big bucks. So they took a gamble on an old opera house in the unfashionable area of West 54th street and spent six weeks and $400,000 transforming the space into a glittering disco paradise. There was a massive raised dance floor to encourage exhibitionism, couches for socialising and secluded areas for more intimate interactions. There was also a semi-circular light display with shooting neon sunbeams, flashing drop-down lights and mirrors that were hit by lasers in a fragmented fairyland of sound and light.

Opening night on 26 April 1977 was a runaway success, with the likes of Cher, Brooke Shields and Margot Hemingway in attendance. But how could Rubell and Schrager maintain this exclusive vibe on a night-to-night basis, avoiding too many bagels (Jews) and bridge-and-tunnel types (commuters)? They decided to implement an arbitrary, Kafkaesque door policy. A nineteen-year-old bouncer who had been schooled in Rubell's standards wielded unlimited power over the desperate throngs vying for entry. They pranced and strutted and donned increasingly outlandish costumes as though on a catwalk. But, unless you were Andy Warhol, Michael Jackson or Truman Capote, it was impossible to predict whether you'd be let in.

Rubell said it was like tossing a salad or baking a cake – you needed an indefinable mixture of people with the right energy. 'Sorry, we don't need any more Eurotrash tonight.' 'Sure, we could do with the McDonald's worker and the limo driver.' 'Rollerina', a woman – reportedly a city lawyer – in roller skates and shorts usually whizzed by. As did a naked bride dubbed 'Maid Marian', her nondescript husband and 'Grandma', a blue-haired woman in her eighties. The wannabes were on tenterhooks as the night dragged on and, despite their kimonos, despite their connections, despite the fact that they'd gone to the club the week before, they were still banned.

The door policy brought out the worst in human nature but it certainly made gaining entry intoxicating, and once you were inside you rejoiced at being one of the chosen. Gorgeous, towering drag queens emerged like butterflies after a day of primping to dazzle and delight, often bewitching hetero men in the process. The bartenders – chosen by Rubell – were sexy, impudent young men who served guests in their underwear and could usually be persuaded to give sexual favours for a price. But the real stars were the DJs who used the club as a testing ground for the soaring disco tracks that would later become mainstream hits. When Gloria Gaynor wanted the B-side of a Righteous Brothers song to get some airtime, she called up Studio 54. The clubbers loved it and soon 'I Will Survive' was the top hit of the year and the iconic disco anthem of all time.

Rubell and Schrager knew that fun doesn't just happen. It takes hard work and planning. Rubell had the vision, Schrager had the organisational skills and, between the two of them, they staged elaborate theatricals that cost tens of thousands of dollars and were dismantled the next day. Theme nights such as 'Disneyland', 'Louis XIV' and 'Grease, the musical' were meticulously carried out – they shipped in vintage automobiles for Grease. The Studio 54 Hallowe'en bash could not be missed. For Dolly Parton's birthday they turned the club into a barn with haystacks and living farm animals. When the designer Halston wanted to throw a party for Bianca Jagger, they imported a white horse. Camera-loving Bianca leapt onto its back for the now classic photograph of the club.

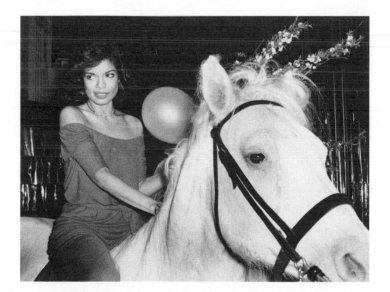

A month after opening, Studio 54 had its liquor licence revoked on a technicality. What should have been a disaster did nothing to dent the crowds or stop the fun since they were all on coke. Cocaine was the social lubricant of Studio 54, the drug that dissolved inhibitions and made everyone feel like a conqueror, the drug that made disco music sound like Mozart and gave them the energy to dance non-stop till sun-up. 'Got any coke?', 'Got any coke?', everyone would ask each other, even if they already had their own. If you could score from an Arab sheik, why not? Users would toss grams of coke at the bartenders or snort it through hundred-dollar bills, discarding them for scavengers to find. The ladies' bathroom, with its adorable pink vanity tables with matching stools and mirrors, was a favourite spot for stylish snorting, as was a special section known as the 'nosebleed room'.

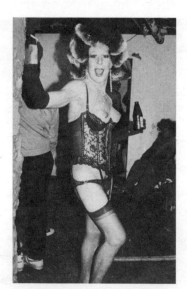

The squalid basement furnished with stained rugs and cushions became the VIP area, where the thudding music from above shook down dust from the filthy ceiling, and once a forgetful bar boy left an Italian princess handcuffed to the exposed piping to be abused by all.

If heroin was the drug of punk, cocaine was the drug of disco. The numbing, warming effects of heroin soothed the angry, nihilistic punks and helped them to forget. But coke users weren't looking for obliteration and instead sought a vivid, wide-awake high. Coke, like disco music, is sexy but impersonal and therefore complemented the fast beats and synthesised voices in the songs.

Studio 54 was full of beautiful people and the coke only made them look and feel better. With Donna Summer's orgasmic moans of 'Love to Love You Baby' pulsing in their veins and an unlimited selection of gorgeous, willing bodies, it's no wonder that coked-up partiers couldn't resist doing each other in situ. Sex was happening everywhere: in the toilets and corridors, under the tables, behind the bar and especially on the balcony coated in black rubber – designed specially so that the semen could be easily hosed off the next day. One woman enjoyed standing on the balcony and being fucked from behind so that she could still admire the dancers. Once, Rubell staged an ejaculation contest for his bartenders, awarding the farthest shooter with a trip to Barbados (with him).

Caution was not a virtue that held much sway at Studio 54. Most STDs could be cured by antibiotics and cocaine wasn't even addictive ... and so they continued with reckless abandon. Rubell and Schrager were raking in the cash, their registers overflowing. In 1977, they paid only $7,000 in tax on £13 million in sales. Rubell was high on Quaaludes and short on discretion. Soon, the scam was common knowledge.

On 14 December 1978, they were busted by the feds, who uncovered evidence in accounting books which had been left lying on a table along with a bag of cocaine. They now faced multiple felonies for tax evasion and drug possession in one of the biggest IRS coups in history. The Feds also found a list, which made it into *New York Magazine*, of all the celebrities who had been given 'party favours' or drugs by the club owners. At the beginning of 1979, Rubell and Schrager pleaded guilty to the escalating charges and managed to get reduced two-year sentences by informing on fellow club owners. It was around this time that Hamilton Jordan, President Carter's Chief of Staff, was investigated for allegedly snorting cocaine at Studio 54.

In February of 1980, the club threw a lavish going-down party for the unrepentant duo, who would be heading for the Metropolitan Correctional Center next day. A ticker-tape banner vilified the IRS and above hung the man in the moon with a cocaine spoon in his mouth. Two songs played on repeat: Frank Sinatra's 'I Did It My Way' and Gloria Gaynor's 'I Will Survive'.

Studio 54 had encouraged a high gay turnout and in the following years many of the old clubbers, Steve Rubell included, came down with a mysterious illness that turned out to be Aids. Not all of its victims were men. In 1992, 26-year-old Ali Gertz, a beautiful, privileged young woman from the Upper East Side – Park Avenue to be precise – died of Aids, having contracted the disease from an uninspiring one-night-stand at Studio 54 as a teenager.

The social phenomenon that was Studio 54 depended on disco, sex and cocaine. Hedonism flamed out with the Aids epidemic and a Technicolor fantasia became black and white, sombre and all too real. The brand Cocaine suffered through association. The drug became linked with violence, disease and death.

3

MIAMI AND COLOMBIA

MIAMI VICE

While Jimmy Carter's drug advisers and the media were not especially worried about cocaine, something curious was happening in south Florida. The region, which had always profited from illicit goods thanks to its unguarded, thousand-mile coastline, had become the cocaine entrepôt of the world. Increasing demand coincided with increasing supply – economic troubles and crop failures had driven Peruvians and Bolivians to grow more coca – and cocaine was entering Florida at an unprecedented rate. This resulted in an explosion of related violence as established Cuban Americans fought turf wars with immigrant Colombians who, no longer content with being distant suppliers, were now trying to take over distribution in the state and beyond.

In the space of few years, the formerly sleepy state turned into the Wild West. The cops, outnumbered and outsmarted, were unable to cope with the scale of the business and had no idea who the major players were in the trade. Drug barons possessed unlimited funds for speed boats, planes, night landings, even parachute drops. Between 1979 and 1981 the murder rate in Miami doubled, far surpassing New York City. Dade County, West Palm Beach and Fort Lauderdale were equally dangerous.

Shoot-outs took place in broad daylight, bodies were turning up in unusual places such as the courthouse men's room. Mostly it was dealers killing other dealers, but if you're using a machine gun there's collateral damage. One notorious murder occurred in July 1979 when a white delivery truck displaying the logo HAPPY TIME COMPLETE PARTY SUPPLY drove into the parking lot of a big Dadeland mall. Several gunmen strolled into a nearby liquor store and comprehensively minced a top Miami trafficker with hundreds of rounds. His body was so mashed it took several days for the police to identify him.

The rapid influx of drug money boosted the Florida economy and in 1979, a time when the national economy was in the doldrums, the Miami Federal Reserve reported a cash surplus of $5.5 billion. Cocaine provided the state with a huge source of revenue, with the black-market economy at an estimated $11 billion. Traffickers were brazenly walking into banks to deposit millions in one transaction. When the government started to enforce the Bank Secrecy Act, which limited single deposits to $10,000 at a time, the dealers hired lackeys to go from bank to bank with suitcases of cash. They invested in front businesses and real estate – mostly paid for in cash – which led to a property boom.

The DEA and federal government moved in with force to impose order. One of the first big-time dealers to catch their attention was Griselda Blanco.

PROFILE: GRISELDA BLANCO (1943–2012)

In 1979, at the age of thirty-six, Griselda Blanco de Trujillo headed the most-wanted list of cocaine traffickers in Miami. She was variously known as the 'Godmother', 'Muñeca' (little doll) and 'Stutterer' (she had a speech impediment), but the nickname that suited her best was 'Black Widow' – because of her habit of mating and killing. All three of her husbands ended up dead, most likely knocked off by her. By the end of her drug reign, she had killed anywhere between forty and 250 people, including a two-year-old boy.

Griselda's rough childhood in Medellín, where she earned a living as a pickpocket, habituated her to a life of drama and crime. Legend has it that at the tender age of eleven she kidnapped a rich child for ransom and then shot him. Young Griselda was attractive – small, voluptuous (later turning to fat), round-faced and dimpled. She had a penchant for hats, turbans and wigs, and bragged about a piece of jewellery that had supposedly belonged to Eva Perón. Griselda's good looks led her to prostitution at fourteen and then to serial marriages from the age of twenty with drug dealers who taught her the trade.

In time Griselda demanded a larger stage than Medellín could provide. In the mid-seventies, she and her second husband, Alberto Bravo, moved to Queens, but their debut into a new world was marred by an indictment in Brooklyn for smuggling 150 kilos of cocaine. They escaped back to Medellín, where they joined the burgeoning community of nouveau riche cocaine dealers. They owned multiple houses and held parties at the Intercontinental Hotel, sometimes inviting all of their cocaine laboratory workers to attend. Already fired up on *aguardiente* when they arrived, these poncho-clad country bumpkins habitually soiled the ballroom with vomit and piss before going after each other with broken bottles and knives. A good time was had by all.

Griselda's marriage to Bravo ended badly when she pulled out a gun from her ostrich-feathered boot and shot him in the face along with several bodyguards during a business altercation in a Medellín parking lot. Although badly injured, the incident did not dampen her spirit and she took her bloodlust with her to Miami, where in the late seventies and early eighties she built her cocaine empire. She enforced discipline with an armed group of thugs called *Los Pistoleros* who used the *sicario* technique of assassination. Blanco is credited with inventing this now-popular method which involves two men on a motorcycle (one drives, the other carries a gun) shooting at a target in a car. During this period Griselda also designed a range of women's underwear with secret compartments for cocaine.

In the infamous 1979 Dadeland shootout, the hitman, Paco Sepulveda, was related to Blanco's third husband, Dario Sepulveda. She and Dario frequently argued over who was a better killer, and named their son Michael Corleone Sepulveda after the character in *The Godfather*. Michael was so precious to Griselda that she reportedly murdered an employee solely for picking the boy up twenty minutes late from the Miami airport. When she separated from Dario, they became embroiled in a bitter custody battle, which naturally was resolved by her husband's murder.

Griselda was not good at taking care of her debts. Instead of paying Marta Ochoa the $1.8 million she owed her, she had her killed and dumped her bullet-infested body into a canal. Such a murder was especially risky given that Marta was the cousin of top trafficker Jorge Ochoa. As a precaution, Griselda relocated to Irvine, California where she employed three sons from her first marriage, Oswaldo, Dixon and Uber. Two of them were murdered in the normal course of her cocaine business.

In February 1985 Griselda was arrested on charges of murder and racketeering. She just avoided the death penalty and spent nearly two decades in jail in Miami and New York. On her release in 2004 she was extradited to Colombia where she attempted to live out a quiet retirement. She had made many enemies over the years. On 3 September 2012, the 69-year-old grandmother was fittingly targeted by a *sicario* while leaving a butcher's store in Medellín carrying over $100 worth of meat. She bled to death on the sidewalk while her ex-daughter-in-law held a Bible over her wounds.

Griselda Blanco is rare for being a successful female trafficker in a male-dominated profession. She defied all stereotypes about feminine timidity and weakness, and might be celebrated as a feminist entrepreneur but for her pathological disregard for human life, along with the law. Griselda has the distinction of being the first drug baron (or rather, baroness) to be studied in any detail by the DEA, which had yet to understand that the real threats were safely conducting their operations from Colombia. Within the next few years, the entire cocaine trade was wholly appropriated by the Medellín cartel.

PROFILE: CARLOS LEHDER (1949–)

Carlos Enrique Lehder was slight (5 ft 6 in. and under 10 stone) but clever, good looking and charismatic. Born to a German father and Colombian mother, he moved to the US from Colombia when he was fifteen and was fluent in both Spanish and English. In 1974, the 25-year-old was sentenced to four years at a minimum security prison in Danbury, Connecticut for smuggling marijuana. This was a propitious internship for the budding criminal because it was in Danbury (which he later referred to as his 'college') that he met a banker who taught him money laundering, a doctor who knew all about extradition treaties and, most importantly, George Jung, a former football player who had made hundreds of thousands of dollars flying marijuana from Mexico into California.

George and Carlos were bunkmates and spent the next year and a half reading classics and pop psychology, weightlifting, discussing politics and strategising about cocaine. In 1974, cocaine, unlike marijuana, was not shipped in bulk. If they could find a means of moving large amounts, they knew they could make a fortune. With Lehder's Colombian contacts and Jung's experience flying dope, they were a perfect match. In 1976, on leaving prison, they set up their practice.

The basis to their success was a limitless appetite for cocaine in Los Angeles. A hairdresser friend of Jung's had many contacts in Hollywood and managed to sell 10 kilos of uncut coke in the space of two weeks. This sale won Lehder instant credibility with drug barons in Colombia, promising a rewarding partnership. Once or twice a week, Jung took the red-eye from Miami to Los Angeles, carrying about 20 kilos and returning with suitcases stuffed with $100 bills. Jung and Lehder each kept $100,000 per trip and sent the rest back to Colombia. Jung frittered his money on women and drugs while Lehder invested his, never touched cocaine and dreamt of expansion.

In August 1977, Lehder hired Barry Kane to fly 270 kilos of cocaine from Colombia to the US, stopping off in the Bahamas to refuel. This successful flight gave Lehder the confidence to build a smuggling haven in the Bahamas – a plan that did not include Jung, who was now addicted to coke and doing as much as 8 grams in one binge. Jung then made the fundamental error of introducing Lehder to his hairdressing contact in California. He realised his mistake when he was cut out of the loop.

Norman's Cay is a small island in the Bahamas

about 200 miles south-east of Miami and therefore a perfect smuggling base. Lehder chose it for its natural harbour and pre-existing airstrip and because it was small enough to take over. He bought up most of the properties, which he paid for in cash, and got rid of all other tenants, including news anchor Walter Cronkite, through bribery or intimidation. Doberman pinschers and German soldiers were brought in to guard the island along with Colombian prostitutes to service his employees. He equipped the island with the latest look-out technology.

Lehder had trouble finding pilots so he enrolled some of the LA hairdresser's friends in flight school. His new pilots, many of whom were drug users, included a disc jockey, a dishwasher and an ex-marine short on his alimony payments. They worked hard, flying hundreds of kilos of cocaine from Colombia to Norman's Cay and then to the United States. Stephen Yakovac, a pilot who kept track of inventories, noted that he had personally shipped 1.5 tons of cocaine into the US during seven trips in 1978. Lehder's fame spread. Pablo Escobar and Jorge Ochoa began paying him to transport their cocaine. On 16 August 1978, 28-year-old Jorge Ochoa landed on Norman's Cay in a plane stuffed with 314 kilos of cocaine, the biggest load to date. Escobar, who used Bahamian banks to store his money, dropped in occasionally to enjoy the island's amenities. Lehder had joined the big league.

At first there was a party atmosphere on Norman's Cay as his hippy employees exulted in their newfound riches and utopian lifestyle. Problems developed when they all began taking too much cocaine, which made them paranoid and addled. Even Lehder, who had previously shunned the drug, was now addicted to base. At night he would maniacally count stacks of bills while holding forth about his political ambitions. His ideology was a mix of neo-Nazism (thanks to his German heritage) and anti-imperialism. He spoke about dismantling America's hegemonic police state with cocaine and saw himself as a charismatic leader whose influence would soon extend across the globe. The 29-year-old had become a messiah.

In the space of a year the beautiful Bahamian island turned into an armed fortress populated by crazed drug addicts. Dozens of daily flights notified the Bahamian authorities that something suspicious was going on and a raid took place in September 1979, which resulted in the imprisonment of Lehder and thirty of his men. It was not difficult to bribe the authorities and the men were promptly released. Bribery kept them out of trouble and cocaine money lined the pockets of many seemingly respectable officials, including, it is said, Prime Minister Pindling, the father of Bahamian independence.

Local government was sorted but the US government proved more rigid. When Lehder was indicted by an American jury in Jacksonville, Florida on 8 January 1981 for smuggling, conspiracy and tax evasion, he became the most wanted drug lord in America. He fled Norman's Cay in September of 1981, but continued supervising his business from afar. The island, which for five years existed as a principality with the highest GDP per capita in the world, was shut down for good in 1984.

After his indictment, Lehder relocated to his hometown of Armenia, Colombia, where he careered around in sports cars, bought up properties and businesses and impregnated a series of local girls, who all developed drug problems. He considered creating a Bavarian-themed shopping complex and erected a seven-foot bronze statue of a nude John Lennon with bullets in his back, the letters 'Peace' on his right hand and an inscription declaring him the greatest musician of all time.

Lehder was still a big player in the Colombian cocaine community but his star was fading. His erratic behaviour, which included airing his Nazi sympathies by blaming 'international Zionism' for problems in Central America and arguing that 'Adolfo' Hitler hadn't been *that* bad, did not lower his profile. The US and Colombian authorities were on his tail. Further, his braggart ways had alienated Escobar, who had come to see him as a US-raised intruder.

By the mid-eighties, Lehder was on the run. In 1985, dressed in army fatigues, he gave an interview for Spanish television from his Colombia hideaway. He expressed his hatred of an America 'guided by *Playboy* magazine' and 'drunk on pornography'. In February 1987 he was captured by the Colombian police in compliance with US extradition laws and flown to America to stand trial. This was the first time that a major cocaine trafficker had been captured. Lawyers compiled a dossier on his illicit activities and the IRS socked him with a $70 million bill after determining that he had earned $300 million between 1979 and 1980 alone. Lehder, convinced that he could beat the system, sent a personal letter to Vice-President George Bush asking for immunity. He received no response.

The trial commenced in November 1987. Witnesses including George Jung and other wronged former friends and lovers were more than happy to testify against the man branded 'the Henry Ford of cocaine transportation, with a mission to destroy the consumer' by the prosecutor. The 38-year-old Lehder, dressed in an incongruous business suit, looked sombre and said nothing. After seven days of deliberations he was convicted on all counts. When brought back for sentencing two months later on 20 July 1988, he had grown a full beard and moustache and, fired up on coke and hubris, held forth eloquently for half an hour without notes. Accusing the court of racism, he denounced the trial as illegal, saying, 'I feel like an Indian in a white man's court.' His performance went unheeded and he was given the maximum sentence of life without parole – he is still working hard from prison to overturn this sentence.

THE MEDELLÍN CARTEL

Medellín is the largest city in Colombia after Bogotá and the capital of the Antioquia province. The men and women of the region are known as *paisas* and pride themselves on their simple strength and determination. Medellín has always been home to illegal entrepreneurs but drug dealers often retired decorously to mansions in the country once they had made enough money to lead a good life. This all changed in the mid-1970s when Medellín became the cocaine capital of the world.

There was lethal competition for control of the burgeoning cocaine trade. Violence rocked the provincial city as would-be drug lords combated for power, enacting reprisals against their enemies. Over forty people were cut down in one weekend in 1975 in what was known as the Medellín massacre. By the late seventies, a handful of successful traffickers merged to form the top rung of the Medellín cartel: Pablo Escobar, José Rodriguez Gacha (aka 'The Mexican'), the Ochoa brothers and, to a certain extent, Carlos Lehder, who, while never fully accepted, was initially needed for his US contacts.

The young Medellín cartel was a loose affiliation of members rather than a strictly hierarchical outfit. In April 1981 the lead players flew their private jets to Hacienda Veracruz, the Ochoa family compound on the Caribbean coast with a bull ring, zoo and man-made island. The purpose of the summit was to discuss expansion. They were avid for more of everything: more planes, more trafficking routes, more cocaine and more money. They discussed their business model, agreeing to share loads, compartmentalise, divvy up jobs and professionalise their enterprise. They could now corner the market.

Later that year, Jorge Ochoa's sister, Marta, was kidnapped

by M-19, a guerrilla group, and held for ransom. Kidnappings were common occurrences in Colombia and M-19 had no idea that they had picked on the wrong target. They were about to witness the full wrath of the newly emboldened Medellín cartel.

The cartel convened a 'general assembly' and created a vigilante group called *Muerte a Secuestradores* (MAS) or 'Death to Kidnappers'. Two hundred and twenty-three drug traffickers donated $20,000 a piece to the cause and notified the public of their existence by dropping flyers over a football stadium. After a brief, bloodthirsty campaign, they captured the leader of M-19 and secured the release of Marta Ochoa on 17 February 1982.

From this moment, the Medellín would have no compunction about using terror tactics to bring the people, the rebel groups and the government of Colombia into submission. Its doyen and de facto leader was Pablo Escobar.

PROFILE: PABLO ESCOBAR (1949–93): PART I

Pablo Escobar, perhaps the greatest criminal of all time, was 5 ft 6 in. and plump, with a double chin, lazy eyes and curly hair. He grew a moustache and dressed casually – his preferred uniform consisted of jeans, polo shirts and white Nikes. His voice was soft and not uneducated (except when he broke into the local slang) and he could be gentle and charming. But his defining feature was his ruthlessness. Anyone who got in Pablo's way was made to meet their maker.

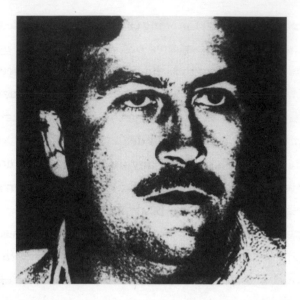

Escobar was born outside of Medellín on 1 December 1949, during *La Violencia*, a period of political upheaval and bloodshed. Legend has it that he was raised in penury but pulled himself up by his criminal bootstraps by robbing tombstones. This story is most likely apocryphal since Pablo's parents were well-to-do and middle class by *paisa* standards. His father was a cattle farmer and his mother, Hermilda, whom he loved and admired unreservedly, was an ambitious teacher who dreamt of great things for her young son. Pablo dropped out of school at sixteen and spent his youth smoking weed, going to bed at 1 or 2 a.m. and waking up late in the afternoon, habits he would maintain for the rest of his life. Cocaine did not agree with him.

Criminality was a norm in Medellín and the city provided young Escobar with opportunities for honing his black-market skills. He became a car thief and earned a reputation for being calm, cheerful and deadly. Instead of paying his dues or networking, like other would-be cocaine barons, he abandoned social niceties and, in 1975, went straight for the jugular by murdering Fabio Restrepo, one of the biggest cocaine traffickers in town. Slick, well-connected dealers such as the Ochoa brothers who hadn't paid any attention to this country thug suddenly changed their attitude. From now onwards, nobody dared cross Pablo Escobar.

Everyone wanted in on the cocaine bandwagon, which boosted the Colombian economy thanks to the influx of American dollars. The line between legitimate and illegitimate business was blurred as otherwise innocent parties invested in shipments of cocaine while the government turned a blind eye. Pablo devised a relatively risk-free insurance policy called *apuntada* which covered lost shipments (at their Colombian rather than US sale price) but he took a 10 per cent cut if they reached their final destination. Everyone made a profit, even if few shipments were intercepted along the way (only about one in ten loads were caught). Those with reservations realised that it was better to work for Pablo rather than get killed. It was a devil's bind: *plato o polmo* (silver or lead), i.e. bribery or death.

The small city of Medellín was overrun by traffickers and their money. They frequented venues such as Las Margaritas, Kevin's and the Intercontinental Hotel, and tried to surpass each other in ostentatious displays of wealth. They rode in limousines, hired bodyguards and procured the most glamorous arm candy. They also bought massive *fincas* or ranches, flying guests in by private jet.

Los Nápoles, Pablo's 7,000-acre *finca*, cost $63 million before he added the artificial lakes, swimming pools (decorated with marble Venuses) and other necessities. Naturally, he needed a zoo – Colombian cocaine barons love zoos – with more than 200 roaming animals including a pair of black cockatoos costing $14,000 each. Pablo, who styled himself as a Chicago-style gangster, mounted a bullet-riddled vintage car on a pedestal, claiming that it had belonged to Al Capone.

He was a fun-loving and generous host. He rented out football stadiums and staged amateur matches with glaring lights and professional announcers. He flew local beauty queens to Los Napoles for his friends' delectation and engaged the women in sexual games, sometimes involving a gynaecological chair. He had a lifelong penchant for girls between fourteen and fifteen years of age although he was devoted to his wife Maria Victoria (fifteen when she married him) and their two children, Juan Pablo and Manuela. He took his and his brothers' families on a memorable trip to the US, going to Disney World in Florida and Graceland in Memphis and on a tour of the White House and FBI headquarters.

Making millions was not enough for Pablo, who also wanted to be revered and loved by the people of Colombia. In 1982, he satisfied a need for public approval by being elected as an alternate representative to the Colombian Congress. He set about winning the hearts of the poor of Medellín by lavishing their children with Christmas presents, building roller-skating rinks and low-income housing, handing out wads of cash and delivering speeches about the inequities of the world. He bought newspapers which churned out Escobar propaganda. One of them hailed him as a Robin Hood of the *paisa*, a heroic reputation he still maintains in certain parts of Colombia.

ENOUGH IS ENOUGH

American cocaine users and Colombian distributors had entered into a mutually beneficial partnership. The street price of coke was falling due to increased supply and the Colombians were still getting rich from the growing volume of sales. But Ronald Reagan, who had become President in 1981, was a screen action man who needed to prove himself in the new role. He took charge of the well-publicised cocaine crisis in Florida, where almost half the murders were drug-related. The DEA went into assault mode, launching Operation Greenback to confiscate illegal assets and setting up 'Centac' – the Central Tactical Unit – to combat traffickers. In January 1982 the government launched an offensive with Vice-President George Bush in command. More than 200 federal employees were sent to Florida with full military support from the US army and navy.

The largest cocaine seizure to date (four times the previous amount) came in March 1982 when nearly 2 tons – worth more than $100 million wholesale – were found by agents inspecting the cargo of a Colombian air transport company.

The scale of the bust was one of the first indicators that the Colombian traffickers were no longer operating as individuals but as part of the Medellín cartel. The DEA, which had been relatively clueless about cocaine manufacturing in Colombia, decided to go after cocaine at its source. For this they would need the cooperation of the Colombian government.

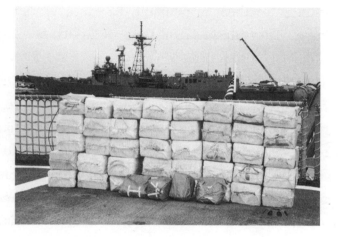

SNOW PATROL

Johnny Phelps, a 6 ft 4 in. red-haired DEA agent from Texas, arrived in Bogotá in 1981, establishing himself as serious irritant to the Medellín cartel. Jaime Ramirez, a razor-sharp Colombian with a detailed grasp of his country, became head of their Anti-Narcotics Unit in 1982. And in 1983, Lewis Tambs, a gruff but charming 55-year-old, became US ambassador to Colombia. These three men led the fight against the cartel until the mid-eighties.

Precursor chemicals, including ether and acetone, are needed to make cocaine. When Phelps realised that large quantities of illegal ether, imported from the US or west

Germany, were going straight through Colombian customs, he began dismantling the network of chemical suppliers. American companies were now expected to report suspicious orders to the DEA. Thus, when a certain Frank Torres tried to buy nearly 2 tons of ether in November 1983, the salesman at the New Jersey chemicals company stalled the order while he contacted the DEA. Here was a rare opportunity for them to pinpoint the exact location of a cocaine lab. They attached radio transmitters to a few barrels of ether and monitored their slow progress via satellite.

In early March 1984, the satellite revealed that the chemicals had stopped somewhere in Colombia's eastern jungle region, a dangerous guerrilla stronghold. Jaime Ramirez's task force was sent in and discovered a giant cocaine lab with an airstrip, kitchen and sleeping quarters to accommodate dozens of employees. A logbook revealed that 15 tons of cocaine paste, mostly from Bolivia, had entered the lab in less than two months. The lab, named *Tranquilandia*, was destroyed by Ramirez's men. *Tranquilandia* was only one of many jungle labs that had sprung up the previous year, producing thousands of kilos of cocaine a month. Ramirez and his men found more and more labs including *Cocalandia*, *Tranquilandia 2* and *El Diamante*. Thirteen tons of cocaine, fourteen labs, five airstrips, seven planes and thousands of drums of ether went up in smoke in the space of a few weeks, costing the cartel $1 billion in assets plus an estimated $12 billion in future revenue.

The jungle busts were a huge coup for both the DEA and the Colombian government. Enough cocaine had been destroyed to dent its flow into the US, causing the first jump in price in years. While Gacha, aka 'the Mexican', had lost the most, the entire cartel had been humiliated and sought revenge.

PROFILE: LARA BONILLA (1946–84)

The election of Belisario Betancur as President of Colombia in 1982 was a disappointment to the DEA because he refused to revive the lapsed US–Colombian extradition treaty. The New Liberals, who had lost out to his Conservative party, were also disappointed. They had campaigned against the widespread acceptance of political donations from drug traffickers and feared that Betancur would not tackle this problem. Betancur was at least obligated to invite some members of the opposition to join his government and in 1983 he nominated the New Liberals politician Lara Bonilla as his minister of justice.

Bonilla, a popular and idealistic 35-year-old, made it his mission to hound the Medellín cartel, denouncing them in public speeches in which he announced that many of Colombia's football teams were funded by traffickers. He did everything to tarnish Pablo Escobar's reputation, dredging up long-forgotten offences such as his 1974 arrest for car theft and 1976 arrest for cocaine trafficking. He showed that Escobar had been responsible for many of the MAS kidnappings and tried to catch Escobar on petty charges such as the illegal importation of wild animals. Bonilla's allegations put an end to Escobar's cherished political ambitions and in January 1984 he resigned from his position in Congress.

Bonilla's efforts were not actively supported by the Betancur government, but with great courage he continued his solo mission. Escobar, who had been determined to do away with him for some time, convened a drug summit and placed a contract on his life. Word of the contract got back to Bonilla, who arranged a transfer to the Colombian embassy in Prague and tried to organise an immediate trip to Texas. Unfortunately, he didn't act quickly enough. On 30 April 1984 Bonilla's Toyota was followed by a Yamaha motorcycle with a Mac-10-wielding *sicario* who fired a volley of bullets into his head. Bonilla was pronounced dead that evening.

Lara Bonilla's death served as a wake-up call to the country. Everyone in Colombia was all too conscious of its internal strife but had hitherto believed that the state was more powerful than the drug cartels. Now they were not so sure. This open act of terrorism compelled Betancur to sign the extradition treaty which would send traffickers to the US. Extradition was the only thing that struck fear into the hearts of the traffickers, who knew that local laws could be compromised but that American justice was an altogether different game.

TO EXTRADITE OR NOT TO EXTRADITE

Los Extraditables was a Medellín-supported vigilante group devoted to overturning the extradition treaty. They embarked on a kidnapping and murdering rampage that successfully scared off most DEA agents and American embassy officials, including Tambs and Phelps, who were not willing to risk the lives of their children and wives for the sake of the War on Drugs. Colombian politicians, judges and their family members now had to travel with armed body-guards at all times. *Los Extraditables* also hired lawyers who tried to declare the treaty unconstitutional. When this didn't work, they changed tactics.

On 6 November 1985, over thirty armed members of *Los Extraditables* stormed the Colombian Palace of Justice, taking 250 employees hostage. The siege lasted twenty-six hours and resulted in the death of ninety-five people, includ-ing the chief justice, half of the Supreme Court and all of the guerrillas. The building was set on fire and most of the traf-fickers' extradition files were lost.

By 1986, the Colombian people were exhausted and scared. Colombia now had the highest murder rate for a country that was not actually at war; the murder rate trebled between 1980 and 1991. In November 1986, the *Extraditables* assassinated Anti-Narcotics Unit head Jaime Ramirez and the next month bumped off a renowned journalist who had spoken out against the violence.

Both politicians and laymen agreed that it would be better to negotiate with the Medellín cartel in order to stop the bloodshed. In December the Supreme Court, bowed down by the year's trials and tribulations, used a minor technicality (it had been signed by an interim President and needed to be re-signed) to declare the extradition treaty unconstitutional. By June 1987, the extradition treaty was officially dead. The Medellín cartel had won.

Not content with their victory, the cartel wanted to ensure

that the treaty stayed dead and buried for the foreseeable future. Escobar, with the help of Gacha, had presidential candidate Luis Galán, a supporter of extradition, assassinated during a campaign speech on 18 August 1989. Escobar then tried to kill Galán's successor, César Gaviria, by bombing Avianca flight HK 1803. Gaviria was not on board but over a hundred Colombians were killed along with two American citizens – something the US did not take lightly.

PABLO ESCOBAR (1949–93): PART II: THE RECKONING

Escobar's public acts of terrorism worried the American government, which was now willing to provide extensive financial and military support to prevent Colombia from turning into a drug state. American aid ballooned during the early nineties. Some went towards establishing incorruptible police units – scarcely a feasible task. *Bloque de Búsqueda*, or Search Bloc, run by Colonel Martinez in Medellín, was devoted solely to capturing Escobar, the Ochoas and Gacha.

Locating Pablo's whereabouts was nearly impossible since ordinary citizens were too terrified to inform on him. Search Bloc asked an American spying organisation called Centra Spike for help. Centra Spike outfitted two Beechcraft planes with $50 million worth of eavesdropping equipment, and they hovered over Medellín intercepting Pablo's phone calls and radio transmissions. These recordings revealed the inner workings of the cartel and demonstrated to the extent to which Pablo Escobar called the shots. When Gacha was captured in December 1989, Pablo behaved like the consummate professional, filling the position and making sure the business didn't suffer from the loss of his second-in-command.

But Pablo was challenged. His cocaine labs were being regularly destroyed and Search Bloc had killed off some of his most trusted associates. He retaliated in kind with a bombing spree that resulted in over twenty murders a day. He then started kidnapping and killing members of Colombia's wealthiest and most well-connected families, the 'oligarchy' as he referred to them. Before long, Colombia's powerful elite were begging President Gaviria to cut a deal with Escobar. This was exactly what he wanted. After years on the run, he needed a safe place to retreat to where he could concentrate on his work and enjoy some home comforts.

Escobar's lawyers oversaw the terms of his surrender and had him safely ensconced in *El Catedral*, which had been specially designed to suit his needs. With its luxurious furnishings, waterbed, Jacuzzi, dance floor and well-stocked bar, it resembled a holiday resort rather than a prison. Pablo could now relax. He received conjugal visits from his wife and local prostitutes and got fat on meals cooked by his personal chef. He kept a full set of the *Godfather* films in his suite and had a photo of Che Guevara on his wall, along with photos of himself dressed up as Pancho Villa and Al Capone. Pablo was obsessed with his legacy and wanted to situate himself in the tradition of outlaws and gangsters. He kept meticulous records, filing his mug shots, indictments and newspaper articles as well as information on the Cali cartel, a rival cartel that was swiftly encroaching on his business.

The entire prison was working for Pablo, who was able to repair his ailing business via a telephone in his cell. Within no time the cartel was once again shipping about 70–80 tons of cocaine to the US each month. In July 1992, upon discovering that he was about to be transferred to a prison with better security, Pablo Escobar escaped – after taking a lawyer of the Ministry of Justice hostage in his cell. Some speculated that Escobar climbed out of an underground passage hidden in the toilet. Others thought that he had dressed up as a woman. The reality was more straightforward. Ignored by 400 soldiers, the most wanted criminal in the world simply walked free.

President Gaviria was deeply humiliated by the escape that had turned his country into an international laughing stock. With allies throughout Colombia, Escobar could move from safe house to safe house undetected for years. To speed the hunt, Gaviria agreed to allow Delta Force, the US army's secret counterterrorism unit, to train the Colombian Search Bloc team in its state-of-the-art techniques.

After sixteen months of aggressive search, Escobar was proving imaginatively wily. He had invented an elaborate system of codes to avoid detection and was micromanaging every stage of his adventure. Telephone recordings revealed an exultant man who showed no signs of stress. Meanwhile, Search Bloc was floundering. Its employees were being systematically killed by Escobar's hitmen. Those who survived were offered million-dollar bribes to switch sides, an offer that several men found too difficult to refuse. Colonel Martinez worried that the outfit was full of Escobar's spies and was obliged to dismiss his entire force and start anew.

In 1993, the emergence of a merciless vigilante group called *Los Pepes* (*Perseguidos por Pablo Escobar*, or People Persecuted by Pablo Escobar) changed everything. They began murdering Escobar's family members and targeting the administrative staff of the Medellín cartel – the lawyers, money launderers, *sicarios* and close associates. Bodies littered Medellín each morning as they bombed his homes, stalked his family and went after his prized possessions, burning down a warehouse full of vintage cars worth $4 million. In the space of a few months *Los Pepes* caused more damage to Pablo Escobar than the government had done in years. Trusted colleagues were jumping ship and his wife and children tried unsuccessfully to escape the country. His empire lay in shreds.

Los Pepes was an unholy alliance of everyone who hated Pablo Escobar and wanted him dead – and very many did. Its core was made up of former cartel members who had turned on their leader and knew his secrets. They consulted Carlos Lehder for additional information and accepted funding from the Cali cartel. Their attacks also seemed to coincide with details intercepted by Search Bloc, a fact that worried both the US and Colombian governments, who wanted no association with a vicious death squad. Secretly, everyone was pleased someone was finally getting the job done.

By the end of 1993, Escobar's sphere of influence had dwindled to his immediate family – whom he was desperate to protect – and he was now communicating solely with his surly sixteen-year-old son Juan Pablo. These conversations were intercepted by Centra Spike and passed on to Search Bloc, who pinpointed him to a row of houses on Street 79 in *Los Olivos*, a middle-class neighbourhood in Medellín.

On 1 December 1993 Escobar celebrated a lonely 44th birthday with wine and a spliff, waking up the next day at noon as usual. Colonel Martinez's son, who was working for Search Bloc, spotted a fat bearded man sitting in a second-storey window. He instantly recognised the criminal who had been eluding his father for nearly three years. The Search Bloc squad came quickly and surrounded the house. Escobar tried to flee over the rooftop but was gunned down, taking shots in his leg, chest and head. He died instantly. 'Viva Colombia, we have just killed Pablo Escobar,' cried the exultant men, who couldn't resist decorating his corpse with a Hitler moustache.

THE DUST SETTLES

So much money and so many lives had been sacrificed in the search for Escobar. But had it really been worth it? The southern-based Cali cartel had benefited from the focus on Escobar. During the hunt, they had forged strong links with the Colombian police, government and military and would maintain these after his death. They had also learnt from the Medellín cartel's mistakes. They did not rely on a single charismatic leader, instead using small independent cells which were less vulnerable to informants and sting operations. They were technologically innovative and deeply enmeshed with the government, donating to the presidential campaign of Ernesto Samper and bribing a large percentage of the Colombian Congress. Following Escobar's death in 1993, they monopolised the Colombian cocaine trade.

The Colombian people had suffered enormously during nearly ten years of violence and did not want to see another decade of brutality at the hands of the Cali. It was clear to both the country's populace and its government that – regardless of principle or US insistence – a deal must be reached with the new cartel. Meanwhile, America was experiencing its own cocaine crisis.

4

THE EIGHTIES: DAYS OF THUNDER

RIDING THE ZEITGEIST

While Pablo Escobar was extending his fiefdom in the early eighties and his Medellín cartel was shipping large cargoes into the US, the American press continued to portray cocaine as a harmless, fun drug for sophisticated party people. In 1981, *Time* magazine put a martini glass full of cocaine on its cover and wrote a text so adulatory that one could almost suppose the writer had taken a few sniffs. 'Cocaine is becoming an all-American drug. Today, in part precisely because it is such an emblem of wealth and status, cocaine is the drug of choice for perhaps millions of solid, conventional and often upwardly mobile citizens.' The article goes on to favour cocaine over other drugs for not being physically addictive, causing lung cancer or turning people into bores.

The idea of a drug that made you scintillating, amusing and driven appealed to the youth of the eighties, who were sick of the soggy pessimism of the seventies and hippy-dippy nonsense of the sixties. They had found a stimulant that suited their post-ideological mood, a guilt-free substance that would encourage their go-getting hedonism and fan the flames of their narcissism. It suited their acquisitive materialism and if they didn't have to worry about unattractive side effects such as overdosing in the bath, all the better.

Timothy Leary agreed that cocaine suited the cultural zeitgeist: 'Obviously, cocaine is the drug of the day. It is well adapted to our times ... It's a drug that causes euphoria, quite pleasant and sparkling, like champagne. You feel powerful, as if you controlled the world – and intelligent, much more than you actually are.' This is the sentiment shared by coked-up Studio 54 clubbers and Wall Street bankers, who used the drug to fuel the relentless pace of dancing or trading. When something seems too good to be true, it usually is. It was only a matter of time before the honeymoon would end.

In music and Hollywood, cocaine had been around for some time and there were a significant number of casualties by the early eighties, but it wasn't until Richard Pryor's freebasing incident and John Belushi's cocaine overdose that America became aware that coke could be a killer.

PROFILE: RICHARD PRYOR (1940–2005)

Richard Pryor was born in Peoria, Illinois in 1940. His father was a pimp and a hustler and his mother was a prostitute. From the age of ten he was raised by his grandmother, a proud brothel owner who disciplined him with switches and did not shield him from the company of tricks and their clients. He was molested by a teenage paedophile and by a Catholic priest.

Pryor was in the army between 1958 and 1960 but spent most of his time locked up after an episode in Germany where he supposedly assaulted a man for mocking Douglas Sirk's *Imitation of Life*, a Technicolor weepie starring Lana Turner as the mother of a mixed-race girl who passes for white.

In the early sixties Pryor, who had always wanted to be a comedian, began performing on the New York club circuit, opening for the likes of Nina Simone, who sometimes held him like a baby before he went on because he was so nervous. At this point, his brand of comedy was relatively clean-cut and palatable to a mainstream white audience. He modelled himself on Bill Cosby, the handsome black crossover comedian.

Pryor eventually grew sick of his hollow, inauthentic routines. In 1967, standing before a white crowd at the Aladdin Hotel in Las Vegas, he decided that he had had enough. 'What the fuck am I doing here,' he mumbled into the microphone, and walked off. He needed to find his voice. In 1969, Pryor moved to Berkeley, California, where he met radical intellectuals and activists such as Huey P. Newton, co-founder of the Black Panthers, and began using cocaine.

Things began to crystallise for Richard Pryor in the early seventies when he adopted an explicit, offensive and confessional style reminiscent of Lenny Bruce. He dug into his difficult past, dredging up deeply personal material that he transformed into comedy gold thanks to his gift for storytelling and distinctive delivery style. He was unabashedly black in his persona and peppered his performances with words like 'motherfucker' or 'nigger'. He addressed topics that even the bravest comedians found unmentionable, like racial inequality and discrimination. Other times, he just got off on being shocking.

In one sketch he spoke of his fear of becoming a dick junkie. 'I sucked a dick ... you can only do it a few times before you get a habit ... I gotta have a dick,' he moaned. He was an adept mimic and would switch between characters like a deranged ventriloquist. One of his most amusing voices was that of the average, uptight, conservative white man who spoke quietly and fucked politely. 'Hello young woman, would it be alright if I inserted my penis into your vagina' etc. etc. The difference between black and white families was a favourite topic. 'What? You didn't give him any pussy?' the black father says to his daughter. 'Even after he spent $35 on you? Get your ass downstairs.'

In 'Is it Something I Said' (1975), Pryor devoted over four minutes to the cocaine: 'I must have snorted up all Peru. I could have bought Peru for all I snorted, given the money up front and had me a piece of property.' Pryor paused for a few deep snorts and added, 'Somebody told me you put it on your dick you can fuck all night ... 600 dollars a day just to get my dick hard.' Snort snort.

There may have been some truth this story. In her memoir, *Foxy: My Life in Three Acts*, Pam Grier visits her surgeon, who tells her about a Beverly Hills epidemic. 'It's a build-up of cocaine residue around the cervix and vagina. You have it. Are you doing drugs?' Pam says no but admits that she's dating Richard Pryor, who they conclude is either dipping his penis into powdered cocaine before sex – a ritual that has she not yet noticed – or worse, snorting so much it has contaminated his semen. The fact that Pam's mouth goes numb after giving him head surely flags *something*. Their relationship did not last.

Pryor, like many cocaine users, never thought that he would get addicted. Naturally, 'I ain't gonna get hooked, not on coke, you can't get hooked on coke. My friends been snorting for fifteen years, they ain't hooked.' By the late seventies, Pryor was addicted to freebasing. On 9 June 1980, during the filming of *Bustin' Loose*, he reportedly set himself on fire with a butane torch that he had been using to cook cocaine base – he blamed it on 151 proof rum. In flames he ran out of his house in Northridge and was taken to the Sherman Oaks Community Hospital and Burn Center, where he was treated for third-degree burns over his entire body.

It was easy to make light of this ridiculous-sounding incident and of course Pryor enjoyed referencing it in future skits. In 'Richard Pryor: Live on the Sunset Strip' (1982), Pryor said that the explosion happened after he dipped a cookie into a glass of low-fat pasteurised milk. But joking aside, the episode did nearly kill him.

A June 1980 article in *People* magazine recounts the hospital's efforts to keep him alive. First they washed him in a whirlpool bath filled with antiseptics. Then they smeared his flesh with creams to fight infection and placed him in a cylindrical chamber that pumped oxygen into his body. Finally, he was operated on to remove fluid from his lungs and scrape away the scales of carbonised tissue covering his body.

Richard Pryor was a prisoner of his addiction for at least fifteen years. It brought out his abusive side and was partly responsible for the demise of several of his marriages – he married seven times to five different women. In 1986, Pryor talked to film critic Gene Siskel about his cocaine problem.

> Drugs may start out fun but they never end fun. The horror they brought me every night and the guilt they brought me every day are what drugs are about ... People think they can handle it. That's a joke. I became a very big star – as big as anyone could want – and I couldn't handle it. I became a drug addict.

Though he had been clean for a year at the time of the interview, he was still haunted by cocaine. 'If you put some base on the table I'd have to leave the room. I couldn't deal with it.'

Cocaine didn't kill Richard Pryor but his torso remained covered in burn scars and his lungs and heart were weakened from inhaling base fumes. He eventually developed MS, which he said stood for 'more shit', and was confined to a wheelchair. He died of a heart attack in Encino, California on 10 December 2005. He was sixty-five years old, which was pretty good considering how he'd lived.

FREEBASING

South Americans had been smoking *pasta básica* (basic paste) for years before freebasing caught on in the US in the seventies. *Pasta básica* is made from mashed coca leaves, gasoline and sulphuric acid and usually inserted into cigarettes. In 1972, a Californian dealer tried smoking ordinary cocaine, which didn't work because of its low melting point. He contacted a chemist friend who figured that cocaine base could be separated from the hydrochloride salt. To do so, he added an alkali and a solvent (ether is now typical) to powdered cocaine, thus creating a chemically distinct and incredibly potent substance that became known as 'freebase'.

Freebasing first took off in Los Angeles (mostly with Hollywood types and dealers) in the early seventies but remained a niche, secretive affair because large amounts of cocaine were needed and the chemical process was complicated and dangerous. The recipe was not in general circulation until underground handbooks explained the process and a cottage industry of freebasing paraphernalia and chemicals sprang up. By 1980, when Pryor set himself alight, a significant portion of cocaine users (10 to 20 per cent) were freebasing and over 300,000 freebase kits had been sold.

The various freebasing techniques had names such as 'The California Clean-Up Method', 'The Spoon Method' and 'The Baking Soda Method' – this latter was also called 'garbage freebase' because, unlike the other methods, it produced an impure, adulterant-laden final product. Although baking soda significantly reduced the purity of the powdered cocaine, the technique had the advantage of being easy, it could be made by simply mixing cocaine with baking soda and water (some add buttermilk) and cooking it over the stove. The result, a hard, rock-like substance that could be smoked in a pipe, was dubbed 'crack' because of the cracking sound it made when heated.

A new product had been discovered. Until now, cocaine had been the expensive indulgence of rich whites. In this ready-made and much cheaper form it could go downmarket.

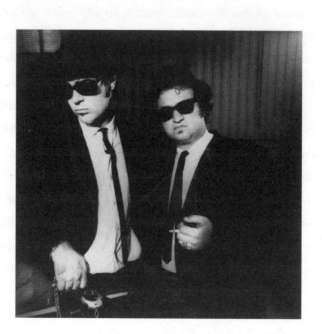

PROFILE: JOHN BELUSHI (1949–82)

John Belushi was born in the Protestant suburb of Wheaton, Illinois to Albanian immigrants. From a young age he saw that humour was his ticket to popularity and had his schoolmates in stitches as the class clown. After high school he made a name for himself at the Second City Comedy Troupe in Chicago and in 1971, when he was twenty-six years old, he was offered a job working for a new comedy series in New York called *Saturday Night Live.*

Saturday Night Live was an immediate triumph and Belushi, along with Dan Aykroyd and Bill Murray, became a household name.

The country was entranced by this lovable dough-ball with chubby cheeks, a cherubic mouth and thick, wildly expressive eyebrows that could ripple with motion or jump out of his head at the slightest provocation. Belushi excelled at physical comedy and impersonations, mimicking everyone from Beethoven to Elizabeth Taylor. He sometimes indulged in method acting and may very well have been on coke when he convulsed his way through an exaggerated rendition of Joe Cocker's 'I get high with a little help from my friends'.

Cocaine use was widespread in comedy circles of the 1970s because it gave performers energy and confidence. Cocaine suited Belushi's driven personality and dedication to excess. He put everything into his work, often pulling all-nighters and spending days on end in the studio. He thought cocaine helped him sustain this frenzied lifestyle. The comedown after the rush of a successful live show was too much for him to bear without the help of stimulants. Cocaine made sure that his high never ended and that the Belushi party kept going round the clock.

In 1978 he stole the show in John Landis's sleeper hit
Animal House, a film that cost $3 million but grossed
over $140 million. It almost singlehandedly invented
the now tired genre of American gross-out comedy with
its simple plot about a group of pimpled, suboptimal
frat boys and their silly antics. Belushi, despite a dearth
of lines, was deemed particularly hilarious as John
'Bluto' Blutarsky. Audiences howled with laughter
when he stuck two pencils up his nostrils or piled up a
gross mountain of food onto his tray at lunchtime. They
loved it when he clapped his hands on his cheeks, spraying boiled eggs onto his classmates and remarking 'I'm a
zit'. A few more iconic moments such as his 'Toga, Toga'
refrain and an inspirational speech with the line 'when
the Germans bombed Pearl Harbor' were enough to seal
his place in comedy history.

By the time Belushi turned thirty in 1979, he had the
No. 1 hit movie with *Animal House* and the No. 1 hit
show with *Saturday Night Live*. It seemed like everything he touched turned to gold. In 1980, he and Dan
Aykroyd had another smash on their hands with *The
Blues Brothers*, a musical comedy film and accompanying album about a paroled convict (Belushi) and his
brother (Aykroyd) who form a blues band to prevent a
Catholic orphanage from closing.

During the filming of *The Blues Brothers*, Belushi's
cocaine addiction became disruptive. Deciding he had
to do something about it, he hired a bodyguard, Smokey
Wendell, to prevent him from coming into contact with
any drugs. Smokey followed him around when he went

to parties, intercepting cocaine and scaring off drug-bearing acquaintances. After eighteen months of being clean, Belushi thought he had beaten his problem and told Smokey he was no longer needed.

Continental Divide, starring John Belushi in his first semi-serious role as a newspaper man investigating a corruption scandal, was released on 18 September 1981 and flopped at the box office. After a lifetime of successes Belushi took this commercial and critical failure badly. He fell off the wagon. He drowned his sorrows in cocaine and alcohol and began mixing with a very unsavoury crowd of addicts and sycophants. One new friend and constant companion, Cathy Evelyn Smith, aka Cathy 'Silverbag' because she doled drugs out of a silver handbag, had been on the fringes of the music world and Hollywood since the sixties, starting out as a groupie and backing singer for 'The Band'. Somebody in the group had fathered a child with her but since nobody knew who – not even Cathy – it was christened 'baby'. Now she dealt drugs to the stars and their acolytes and was usually wasted herself.

On 3 March 1982, Belushi's agent gave him $1,000 to buy a guitar from Guitar Center. Instead, he called up Cathy Smith and bought drugs. That evening Belushi, Smith and an SNL writer went on a bender. They dropped in on various joints in West Hollywood before entering On the Rox, the VIP section of the Roxy. By the end of the night Belushi was so out of it that Cathy drove them back to Bungalow 3 at the Chateau Marmont on Sunset Boulevard. After puking, he felt well enough to snort some more cocaine and receive visitors. Between 3 and 4 a.m. Robin Williams and Robert De Niro dropped by separately for about half an hour each. Williams snorted a few lines of coke. Neither man stuck around, because the atmosphere seemed a little too creepy and Cathy was a 'lowlife'.

The remaining details of the night are hazy but at some point Cathy injected Belushi with a mixture of cocaine and heroin – a speedball – because he was afraid of needles and didn't want to do it himself. She put him in the shower, helped him into bed and turned on the heat when he complained of the cold. Despite noting that he was 'breathing funny' she failed to call a doctor and instead drove off in his black Mercedes.

At 12:30 p.m. on 5 March 1982, Belushi's martial arts trainer found him lying on his side amongst twisted sheets in a foetal position. Half of his body was dark purple in colour and his tongue was sticking out of his mouth like a gargoyle. At 12:45 an ambulance arrived but he was pronounced dead at the scene. He was thirty-three years old.

John Belushi's death stunned the nation and alerted cocaine-using comedians that the drug was not funny. Cathy Smith initially walked away without any charges. Stupidly, she accepted $15,000 to give an interview to the *National Enquirer* where she admitted that she had been inadvertently responsible. This led to charges of murder for the administration of cocaine and heroin. After several years on the run she was extradited to the United States from Canada and spent fifteen months in prison.

PROFILE: BELINDA CARLISLE (1958—)

Belinda Carlisle grew up in the Thousand Oaks, California with her mother, a stepfather she didn't like and six other siblings – her real father, a travelling vacuum salesman, had hit the road for good. Since her home life didn't have much to recommend it, she focused on a couple of extracurricular activities in high school: cheerleading and shoplifting. Then she discovered punk music.

The punk scene in LA provided refuge to misfits all and sundry, irrespective of musical talent. Anyone could start a band, even if they just slouched on stage looking surly. Belinda experimented with a couple of groups until she and some girlfriends formed an all-female band called the Go-Go's. The Go-Go's put in some hard years, at one point touring with a British ska band in rough cities like Liverpool and Birmingham where they were spat at by ruffians. When they started becoming popular, they lost many of their punk followers who equated success with selling out.

The Go-Go's hit the big time in 1981 with their hit single 'Our Lips are Sealed', an infectious bubblegum confection with an accompanying music video of five bouncy, unconventional girls with crazy hairdos and big grins, driving around in LA and splashing in a fountain. Even though they were kind of badass with their ripped dresses and 'I'll do whatever I want' looks, there was also something touchingly innocent and suburban about them. Belinda was adorable with pretty features and a childishly round face – she struggled with her weight for years.

The Go-Go's weren't your run-of-the-mill girl group since they actually wrote their own songs and played musical instruments – a female drummer is still novel. In the space of three years they sold over 7 million albums thanks to songs such as 'Vacation' and 'Head Over Heels', becoming one of the most successful female groups of all time.

The early eighties were a fun time and the girls were partying hard and keeping up with the boys. For Belinda, this meant a lot of cocaine. She began taking it in the mid-seventies when it was still very expensive. 'I loved it from the first time I did it. And I thought, one day when I can afford this I will buy loads of it, and I did,' she told a reporter in 2010.

By the time the Go-Go's disbanded in 1985, Carlisle's addiction was in full swing and two of her former band-mates had serious drug problems as well. Her habit didn't get in the way of her blossoming solo career and in 1987 she came out with the smash hit 'Heaven is a Place on Earth', a full-blown pop power ballad. She had ditched her punk roots and had grown her hair long. In the video she wore a black, off-the-shoulder dress with a red carnation and clung onto a hunky man in the style of a romance novel cover. A number of equally cheesy hits followed and she seemed like the apotheosis of a 1980s prom queen.

Belinda was piling on the cocaine powder along with the sentimentality, but nobody seemed to notice. Even though she snorted more than most addicts, she was left alone by the media, which only paid attention to train wrecks. In their eyes she had it all. She was beautiful, successful and happily married. All this was true but she also had an eating disorder and a drug problem that she didn't beat until 2005, when, after a three-day drug binge in her London hotel room, she finally decided to seek help. Belinda Carlisle had apparently snorted cocaine every day for thirty years – except for nine months during her pregnancy.

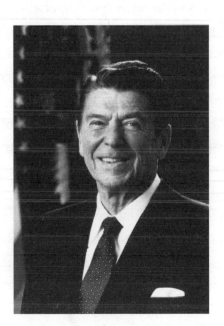

PROFILE: RONALD REAGAN (1911–2004)

Ronald Reagan was sixty-nine years old when he assumed office on 20 January 1981. Despite being the oldest President to date, he exuded confidence and

dependability as well as folksy, all-American charm –
perhaps thanks to his persuasive radio-trained voice
and Hollywood demeanour. Here was a man who the
nation hoped would rescue America from the doldrums
of the 1970s and restore the nation's sense of self.

Reaganites argue that this is precisely what he did
and that his policies were responsible for America's
most boomingly successful decade, the 1980s. Reagan
is an icon of the American right and is credited with
starting America's so-called conservative revolution,
thanks to his supply-side economics which aimed at
cutting taxes and governmental spending in order to
trigger economic growth and clamp down on inflation.
Liberals, meanwhile, claim that his tax cuts only benefited the rich and that government expenditure actually
skyrocketed during his tenure as President.

Reagan certainly funnelled a vast amount of money
into fighting drugs. After the ineffective drug policies of
Ford and Carter, Reagan looked to the hard-nosed Nixon
for inspiration. Nixon had hated drugs but Reagan hated
them even more. And when the Republicans gained
control of the Senate he persuaded them to sanction the
formation of CENTAC 26, a military task force to patrol
the Florida border and combat cocaine smuggling. This
was just the beginning.

On 24 June 1982, Reagan stood in the Rose Garden
of the White House and reaffirmed his War on Drugs –
now the longest war in American history. 'We're taking
down the surrender flag ... We're running up the battle
flag. We can fight the drug problem, and we can win,' he

declared. Nancy Reagan got in on the act, proving a tireless and tiresome spokeswoman in her 'Just Say No' campaign. Most American children of the eighties remember the DARE (Drug Abuse Resistance Education) officers with a mixture of mirth and nostalgia, remarking that these sermons had little impact on their future drug use.

Because actions speak louder than words, Reagan and seventy-eight White House employees peed into bottles and had themselves drug tested in November 1986. A few years later, President George Bush dangled a bag of crack in front of television reporters. Both men had learnt the importance of theatrical high jinks for drumming up public support.

Reagan's anti-drug rhetoric and the younger George Bush's anti-terrorist malapropisms were similarly Manichean. Both spoke of good versus evil, black versus white and us versus them. You either supported American values of freedom and democracy or you didn't. 'Let us not forget who we are,' Reagan urged the nation. 'Drug abuse is a repudiation of everything America is.' He compared the War on Drugs to the Second World War.

Scare stories in the mainstream media did effect some changes. In 1985, 54 per cent of Americans thought drugs, rather than the economy or war, were the biggest threat facing the nation. And there was little resistance to the passage of Reagan's $1.6 billion Anti-Drug Abuse Act in October 1986. Prison capacities would now be expanded and minor drug offenders could be incarcerated for years on end.

Despite Reagan's unflagging efforts, which included a series of large-scale cocaine seizures, the price of cocaine dropped and purity levels doubled during his presidency. While a gram purchased on the street had cost $600 in 1982, the price fell to $200 in 1988. Meanwhile, marijuana prices soared (thanks to continued crop spraying) and many users abandoned pot for cocaine, turning the latter into the youthful drug of choice for the first time ever. Powdered coke and crack use reached unprecedented levels during the 1980s. Cocaine was unquestionably the drug of the decade.

THE DEA REVISITED

In Notorious BIG's posthumous 1997 classic 'Mo Money Mo Problems' he raps about 'No info for the DEA / Federal agents mad cause I'm flagrant / Tap my cell and the phone in the basement'. His rival Tupac shows similar concerns in 'Picture Me Rollin': 'The federales wanna see me dead / niggaz put prices on my head.' By the late eighties and throughout the nineties, the DEA was a source of terror in poor black neighbourhoods. Its SWAT teams wore combat gear and usually chose around 6 a.m. to smash the door and burst in, yelling and waving weapons. The agency was no longer restricted to a deskbound herd of bureaucrats. It had mobilised storm troopers.

Reagan was responsible for turning the DEA into a militarised fighting force by infusing its budget with cash. In 1989, DEA headquarters moved from DC to a more appropriate location across the street from the Pentagon in Arlington,

Virginia. The move made sense, enabling the Defense Department to share its resources, military technology and equipment with the DEA.

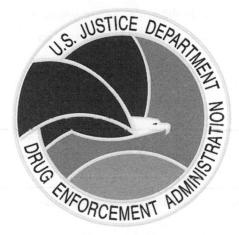

Today the DEA has tens of thousands of employees, nearly 5,500 Special Agents and a budget of $2.2 billion – up from $75 million in 1973. The Special Agents are subjected to an intensive training programme that lasts nearly five months. There are offices and agents deployed around the world. The DEA possesses its own airborne division and a museum celebrating its forty-year history. Beyond being an army, it is an all-American institution.

PROFILE: COCAINE IN LITERATURE

To many non-Reaganites, the 1980s represented the triumph of unfettered, free market capitalism and rampant individualism at the expense of human decency.

The cultural climate depicted in film and literature was one of superficiality and hedonism, with New York at its epicentre. This paradise for the rich and sewer for the poor serves as the backdrop to Oliver Stone's *Wall Street* (1987), a film that, through the amoral exploits of arch-capitalist Gordon Gekko (Michael Douglas), criticises the soulless, money-grubbing values of bankers who live in penthouses, sleep with hookers and snort cocaine.

Coke is ubiquitous in three well-known novels about New York in the 1980s: *Bright Lights, Big City* (1984) by Jay McInerney, *Bad News* (1992) by Edward St Aubyn and *American Psycho* (1991) by Bret Easton Ellis. Cocaine is the blood that pumps through the arteries of the city that never sleeps. It promises glitter and glamour but may very well turn pitiless and mocking. The first two books feature a male anti-hero in his early to mid-twenties who, despite his gilded circumstances, descends into an inferno of drug-induced misery.

The unnamed 24-year-old narrator in *Bright Lights, Big City* is the most sympathetic of the two. Even though he gets fired from his sinecure job as a fact checker at an important magazine (probably the *New Yorker*), we later learn that he is grieving the death of his mother and the departure of his Midwestern model wife who has outgrown him. This may or may not excuse his self-indulgent cocaine binges.

Our narrator's day, until he gets fired, is spent in pre-computer fact-checking land with piles of reference books and an evil spinster boss. At night, he fraternises with a friend who is 'shallow and dangerous, spoilt and rich' but who dangles beautiful, unattainable women before him – women whose fathers are oil tycoons and who live on diets of champagne and caviar on the Upper East Side. Our narrator would like to be part of the tennis-playing, croissant-eating, blue-blooded elite but somehow he always ends up at places called the Lizard Lounger or the Heartbreak club at 6 a.m. with girls with shaven heads and New Jersey accents. Maybe the coke is to blame.

Our narrator is very partial to a little Bolivian Marching Powder, as he calls it. By the end of the night he feels that his brain 'is composed of brigades of Bolivian soldiers. They are tired and muddy from their long march through the night. There are holes in their boots and they are hungry. They need to be fed.' The bathroom with discreet blacked-out windows provides refuge for all weary sniffers and, after a few spoons, he is soaring in the Andean peaks. The high does not last long and he begins to dread the grim, derelict city inhabited by homeless people and drunks. This is the life of a middle-class boy on a cocaine bender.

Patrick Melrose, main character in Edward St Aubyn's five-part series, comes to New York in the 1980s to fetch his father's ashes. This is the father who raped him as a small child, a fact that may have turned him into a cruel bastard and a raging drug addict by his early twenties. Luckily, he is a stinking rich toff who can afford to blow his inheritance on coke, heroin, speed, Quaaludes or whatever drugs he can get can get from his New York dealer Pierre, a man who spent eight years in a mental asylum thinking he was an egg. Or when

Pierre is asleep, he takes a cab past Tomkins Square and Alphabet City until he reaches 8th Street and tries to find some himself. A series of awful escapades ensues.

Melrose makes good use of the withering wit and malice that only an Englishman of his pedigree could possess. Striding around New York with his money, his cut-glass accent and his distinguished good looks, he is wont to irritate even the most benign of readers. And yet, there is nothing sexy about Melrose's addiction, which dominates his waking hours – even causing phantasmal hallucinations. Injected cocaine is not Melrose's only drug of choice but it is a favourite, especially when tempered with heroin. One passage from *Bad News* vividly describes the power of cocaine on the narrator, who smells its 'heartbreaking fragrance' before 'its cold geometric flowers broke out everywhere and carpeted the surface of his inner vision'. St Aubyn compares the act of injecting to being 'drunk on pleasure' and 'choking with love' but also shows the horrors of coming down. When the high subsides, he is 'like a surfer who shoots out of a tube of furling, glistening sea only to peter out and fall among the breaking waves', or he feels 'as if his wings had melted in that burst of light' and he can do nothing but fall. The only option is to start the process all over again.

The physical nature of addiction is conveyed so brilliantly that *Bad News* is one of the most compelling accounts of drug use in literature. It is not so much a novel about the eighties as it is a novel about addiction. In Bret Easton Ellis's *American Psycho*, drug use is a symptom of a deeper problem for a society that has lost its moral compass.

Patrick Bateman, the 26-year-old narrator (an unreliable one since the book switches from first to third person), is a Harvard graduate who knows his own worth. 'I'm creative, I'm young, unscrupulous, highly motivated, highly skilled. In essence what I'm saying is that society cannot afford to lose me. I'm an asset,' he says in the first chapter. These are the characteristics that seem to be rewarded by 1980s corporate America and, in the case of Bateman, they also go hand in hand with a total lack of human empathy. Later, he admits that he 'does not have a single clear, identifiable emotion, except for greed and disgust'. In fact, as the title of the book reveals, Bateman is a psychopath.

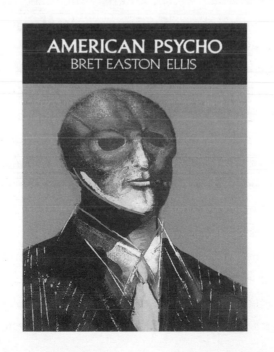

Before we learn about Bateman's blood lust, carried out in a series of psychosexual murders, we get to know his tastes and predilections. His body is a temple that must be worked out, sheathed in expensive clothes, and moisturised, pummelled and pampered to perfection. Since his interior is empty, his exterior is of supreme importance to him. Like a computer or an automaton, Bateman has a photographic memory and a mind for data. Consequently, he loves lists – lists of high-tech technology (now hilariously out of date), lists of expensive food such as 'quail sashimi with grilled brioche and the baby soft-shell crabs with grape jelly' and lists of designer clothes. He occasionally likes to regale the reader with his personal take on the music of 1980s pop stars such as Whitney Houston.

Every man or woman Bateman meets is physically deconstructed. Women, if they are deemed fuckable, are praised for being 'hardbodies' with great asses, big tits, high-heels and designer clothes. He will look at one and do a quick mental assessment: 'Blonde, big tits, wearing a metal-studded dress by Giorgio di Sant'Angelo,' for example. Men cannot get away with being slouches and their clothes are equally important. 'McDermott's got on this wool suit by Lubiam with a linen pocket square by Ashear Bros., a Ralph Lauren cotton shirt and a silk tie by Christian Dior and he's about to toss a coin to see which one of us is going downstairs to fetch the Bolivian Marching Powder.'

Cocaine use amongst the Wall Street types and starlets in Bateman's circle appears to be chronic. In the unisex bathroom of a club called Chernoble everything is quiet except for the sound of sniffing. Sometimes fights break out, perhaps because the coke is too weak, cut with too many additives. These highly stressed types need it to take the edge off. It loosens them up and serves as an aphrodisiac. Many of Bateman's conquests are on coke. In one typically violent scene a girl narrowly misses being murdered by Bateman because she is so high. Alison is a girl Bateman 'did last spring' when he was attending the Kentucky Derby with his girlfriend and her parents. After bedding the very drunk and coke-filled victim, who is presumably unaware of his sexual predilections, he tries to shove his arm, 'gloved and slathered with Vaseline, toothpaste, anything I could find, up her vagina'. This, along with the wire he ties her up with and the duct tape that he straps over her mouth and breasts, is merely a taster of the brutality that is about to follow. The girl is dead meat and he will enjoy watching her bleed to death. And yet, he lets this one get away. Why? He doesn't really know, but thinks it is because she was so high and because she didn't cry. Instead she just moaned 'oh my God' while blood poured out of her nose.

Analysed as an individual, Patrick Bateman is a maniac who ought to be sectioned or imprisoned. But it is perhaps more useful to see him as an exaggerated stand-in for America in the 1980s: a limitless, hubristic society that, drunk on its own power, has forsaken humility. It is no accident that the theory of postmodernism, the idea that there is no centre, that everything is sheen and surface, that reality is a construct or a simulacrum and that life is mediated through technology, really took off during this decade. *American Psycho*, which was lambasted by some critics for its gratuitous violence, was also heralded as a postmodern masterpiece.

THE IRAN–CONTRA AFFAIR

The spectre of communism was very real to Ronald Reagan, who made combating the reds a top priority, even if it meant supporting anti-communist insurgencies. One of his favourite rebel groups, the Nicaraguan Contras, were engaged in a war with the left-wing Sandinista regime, which in 1979 had overthrown an American-backed dictatorship. Reagan was so enamoured of the Contras that he called them 'the moral equivalent of our Founding Fathers' and wanted to do anything he could for them. Unfortunately, the Democrats felt differently and when they assumed control of Congress in 1982, they limited governmental aid to the Contras. Reagan was furious and willing to flout the rule of law to help them. He eventually found the perfect means of doing so.

Since 1980 Iran had been fighting off Iraq and wanted to buy weapons from the US. Reagan, with the support of the CIA, covertly sanctioned the shipment of over 1,500 missiles to Iran despite a governmental embargo. He thought it would relieve tensions with Lebanon – he was willing to exchange arms for hostages – but also hoped to divert the proceeds to fund the Nicaraguan Contras without appearing to do so.

The Iran–Contra scandal broke in November of 1986 after

the Fat Lady, a CIA-owned plane bearing weapons for the Contras, was shot down in Nicaragua by the Sandinistas. The scandal embarrassed Reagan but the bulk of the blame fell on Colonel Oliver North who was in charge of operations, and on the CIA. In the interim, Reagan persuaded Congress to sign a $100 million aid package for the Contras.

DEATH COMES TO AN INVESTIGATIVE REPORTER

The Contra affair is still veiled in mystery, especially in respect of the accusation that the CIA endorsed the Contras' trafficking of cocaine, even allowing them to use planes that had carried weapons into Nicaragua to return to the US laden with the drug.

One of the few people to address this covert governmental sanctioning of drug abuse was Gary Webb, a reporter for the *San Jose Mercury News* who recounted the way in which the CIA-backed Contras sold cocaine to the US in order to use the profits to support their movement. Webb argued that a California dealer, 'Freeway' Ricky Ross, got his coke very cheaply from Nicaraguan drug runner Danilo Blandón who in turn was working for Norwin Meneses, a man in charge of raising US funds for the Contras. The implication of Webb's findings is that the US government, by allowing the Contras to flood the US with cocaine, was indirectly responsible for the crack epidemic despite their purported war on drugs.

Gary Webb's allegations were dismissed by reputable newspapers including the *New York Times* and the *Los Angeles Times* and he was forced to resign from his post. His career was over and he shot himself dead in 2004. It is increasingly acknowledged that there was truth to his findings.

PROFILE: RICKY 'FREEWAY' ROSS (1960–)

Ricky Donnell Ross was born in Troup, Texas but moved to South Central LA as a child. The nickname 'Freeway' was in reference to time spent hanging out under a freeway overpass and his later acquisition of property in the Harbor Freeway area. Ross was a talented athlete and nearly won a scholarship to UCLA, but it turned out that he was illiterate. This made academic success unlikely so he dropped out of Dorsey High School as well as LA Trade Tech, and made money stealing cars and selling their parts.

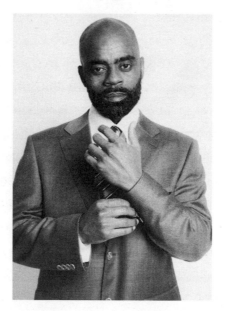

The 1972 hit film *Super Fly*, about a down-on-his-luck cocaine dealer who decides to make one last big deal before quitting the dangerous profession, was Ross's first introduction to the drug. It wasn't until 1979, when a friend gave him coke to sell on his behalf, that the nineteen-year-old Ross realised the money that could be made from selling to a poorer but wider market – cocaine had previously been seen as a niche drug for the rich.

Ross found a reliable coke source, Oscar Danilo Blandón, a Nicaraguan dealer with a wealth of high-quality cocaine (see p. 153). It is unlikely that he knew of Blandón's relationship with the Nicaraguan Contras. Ross started distributing cocaine in Compton with some help from the Bloods and Crips gang members. Within a few years Ross was at the centre of a Los Angeles cocaine ring.

In 1983, Ross began playing around in his kitchen, cooking up 'Ready Rocks', or ready-to-use freebase that could be easily smoked and sold cheaply. In other words, he was making crack. By adding an anaesthetic called procaine he was able to 'blow up' the powder and treble the batches in size, thus trebling his profits. What had started out as an afterthought became his core business and his little rocks sold all over the ghetto and beyond. He had to buy warehouses with supersized vats to accommodate his messy brew but that was no problem now that he making a couple of million bucks a day on crack alone.

Ricky wasn't losing any sleep at night over the scourge that he was inflicting upon his black brothers – let alone the sisters who he was helping turn into crack whores. He didn't even know about all that yet. No one did and wouldn't for at least three more years. Later, Ross would grow to repent his contribution to the crack epidemic, but for now he was enjoying his millions and boy, was he raking it in. In 1984 he was selling about 100 kilos of cocaine a week and by the end of his career he is thought to have made over $600 million. Spending all that money was no easy feat.

How many houses did Ross own? At least thirty but it was impossible to say. His favourite, a neo-classical mansion in Inglewood on Hillcrest Avenue, was purchased for $250,000 and paid for in $1 bills – a favour to its liquor store owner who sold it to him and wanted small notes. Ross also bought up motels and apartment buildings. His mother and girlfriend were sumptuously looked after and given very hefty weekly allowances. There were other women as well ... Ross fathered at least seven children by four different women. Of course he was going to lead a good life, cruising in the hood and partying with Snoop Dogg and the President of Hostess Brands Inc. – the now defunct company that made revolting but iconic American snacks, most famously those taxicab-yellow, cream-filled sponge lozenges called Twinkies.

Ross was both focused and creative. He set up multiple front businesses like his 'shop' on 74th and Western where he sold tyres, or his car wash, his beauty parlour and his motel, a meeting place for dealers called the Freeway Motor Inn. He spent some of his money on cars, designer clothes, holiday resorts and Lakers tickets.

With thousands of employees in southern California, he thought it important to offer compensation and provide legal advice. Everything ran like clockwork under his fierce watch and with the help of state-of-the-art surveillance equipment provided by Blandón which enabled him to cover his tracks and avoid detection. He could offer a bespoke service to important clients, lowering prices when it suited him thanks to Blandón's copious supplies. It was in this way that he blew his competition out of the water.

Los Angeles was swimming in cocaine by the mid-eighties and the market had plateaued. It was time to expand eastward. During the next few years, Ross's tentacles spread from Seattle to St Louis to Detroit, sprinkling crack like a fairy godmother to inner cities throughout the country. Such a large-scale operation could not elude the police forever and Ross had already had a very good run. By investigating Blandón's activities, they were led to Ross and created a task force to track him down. Ross tried to stay out of the game for a while and ruminate on his sins now that the damage he had caused through addiction was becoming apparent even to him. But he loved to work and could always be persuaded to make one last deal.

Ross was caught by a SWAT team in November of 1989 and given a reduced sentence of ten years after pleading guilty. He was out of jail after four years for good behaviour and was welcomed by the community as a figure of redemption. He appeared on television and spoke about the abandoned church that he would turn into a rehabilitation centre. He had the support of the public, large corporations, and celebrities including Magic Johnson and his old pal Snoop Dogg. There was even a book deal and a film contract in the works. Unfortunately, the CIA doubted this about-face and set up a sting with the help of Blandón, who was now a DEA informant. At first Ross didn't take the bait, saying that he wanted to stay clean but he eventually gave in and walked straight into the arms of the law.

Ross was sentenced to life in prison but was released in May 2009. He is now running a social networking site called freewayenterprise.com, working with at-risk children and trying to bring multiple projects into fruition such as a reality TV show and a modelling agency. He also sells human hair from India to women in LA to make a bit of money now that all of his assets have been seized. He is looking forward to a lucrative film deal.

CRACK

Crack arrived in the Caribbean in the late seventies and from there was smuggled to Miami and then to New York by Jamaican gangs or 'posses'. In Los Angeles, the Bloods and the Crips, with the help of Ricky Ross, took care of distribution. This effective bi-coastal marketing ensured that crack had infiltrated large cities like New York, Los Angeles, Miami and Houston by the mid-eighties.

A glut of cocaine in South America ensured that prices continued to drop, dipping sharply after the summer of

1984. One gram of cocaine can generate dozens of crack rocks which were sold for as little as $3. Thus, a seller could make nearly three times what he paid for the powder and find himself a group of reliable customers who would keep coming back for more. Crack became known as the fast food of cocaine and was targeted at the masses.

Crack is highly addictive, so addictive that even animals are enthralled by it. Lab rats crave crack even more than heroin and, in the 1970s, Dr Ronald Siegel, a cocaine expert at UCLA, experimented on rhesus monkeys, which took to smoking crack of their own accord while other drugs required incentives. Crack is rapidly absorbed by the capillaries in the lungs (a surface area much larger than the nose) which can take in unlimited quantities of the drug.

Crack travels directly to the brain rather than entering the circulatory system and within ten seconds the user experiences an intense and euphoric high that wears off very quickly, leaving him feeling depleted, craving another hit. Users can binge on crack for days on end, forgoing sleep, food and any other bodily needs.

CRACK AND INNER CITIES

Why were poor black communities particularly susceptible to crack? Some historians argue that the upheavals of the previous decades – deindustrialisation and the loss of jobs, black middle-class flight to the suburbs, a proliferation of teenage pregnancies and the breakdown of the family unit – resulted in a concentration of vulnerable people who were seeking to dull their pain in a momentary high. And when crack came on the scene it seemed a means of lifting unemployed, disenfranchised men out of poverty and turning them into fledgling entrepreneurs.

A generation of low-level hustlers turned formerly safe parks and playgrounds into no-go areas as drug dealing moved from the periphery to the centre of cities. Turf wars erupted and addicts broke into homes to fuel their habits. Many neighbourhoods went into lockdown. The whites and richer blacks moved out and children were no longer allowed to play in the streets.

In the past, drug addicts were predominately male, but now surprisingly high numbers of women were becoming crack addicts. Many of them came from broken homes, had incomplete educations, were abused as children and gave birth as teenagers. Crack addicts will neglect their own offspring in their all-encompassing cycle of searching and binging. These children were taken into care or looked after by their grandmothers (who were often only in their thirties or forties).

CRACK WHORE

The age-old profession has had many incarnations. Crack, however, was unique in its capacity to generate a new breed of prostitutes who exchanged sex directly for crack rather than money. Crack does not heighten desire but it does loosen inhibitions, which leads to reckless, unprotected promiscuity. But 'crack whores' – the derogatory term designated for them – were desperately in pursuit of crack rather than pleasure. After they had sold all of their material possessions, they turned to their last remaining commodity: their bodies.

All commodities are worth more in times of scarcity. Sadly, this influx of cheap flesh into the market lowered prices, even for non-addicted prostitutes. It robbed the profession of any dignity it might have had since women were now expected to perform any type of sexual act, irrespective of how demeaning it was. 'New girls' experienced a honeymoon phase but their moment of glory was brief. A woman's value decreased with time and she was treated like used goods once she had been on the circuit for too long. The prices she could fetch plummeted just as her hunger for crack increased.

CRACK DEN

Some crack whores went on 'ho strolls' in raunchy attire in order to pick up men. Others lounged around in 'crack houses' or 'crack dens' and waited for men to come to them. The crack den was a designated place for 'geeking and freaking', or taking crack and having sex. This multi-purpose zone of crack-related activity enabled users to buy, sell and use crack or to exchange sex for crack. One witness describes a typical crack den: 'One room they be having sex. Another room they be freaking, like standing on the table, butt naked, dancing. Another room, they be fucking and sucking. Another room, they be smoking.'

Crack dens were often operated out of an addict's home. Generally, he or she oversaw operations and set forth house rules that users were expected to obey. Sometimes there was a cover charge but usually users were simply expected to purchase drugs. The crack house had a social aspect since it facilitated the assemblage of people with a common interest. Male users could chew the fat, bandy drug-related slang, bond over pipe-smoking rituals and satisfy their particular taste at hand.

Full-blown orgies and sex acts of a violent and sadistic nature were not uncommon and sex could last for hours since crack users have trouble achieving orgasm. Men who had felt powerless in the real world found a new arena in which to dominate, cock and crow. Women were automatically expected to provide sexual favours to all, while men weren't.

The crack den often employed a 'house girl' who lived in the house rent-free and was given unlimited supplies of crack for providing unlimited sex. James Inciardi and colleagues document this in a 1993 study:

Upon entering a room in the rear of the crack house (what I later learned was called a freak room), I observed what appeared to be the gang-rape of an unconscious child. Emaciated, seemingly comatose, and likely no older than fourteen or fifteen years of age, she was lying spread-eagled on a filthy mattress while four men in succession had vaginal intercourse with her ... She opened her eyes and looked about to see if anyone was waiting. When she realized that our purpose there was not for sex, she wiped her groin with a ragged beach towel, covered herself with half of a tattered sheet (affecting a somewhat peculiar sense of modesty), and rolled over in an attempt to sleep. Almost immediately, she was disturbed by the door man, who brought a customer for oral sex. He just walked up to her with an erect penis in his hand, said nothing to her, and she proceeded to oblige him...

THE CRACK SCARE

An obscure South Central newspaper, the *Los Angeles Sentinel*, wrote about 'rock houses' as early as 1983. *New York Times* journalist Donna Boundy was one of the first to use the term 'crack', in a 1985 article on drug-addicted teenagers. The story took off and in 1986 and 1987 alone over 1,000 apocalyptic articles on crack had been published in major US newspapers and magazines.

In June 1986, *Newsweek* published 'The Plague Among Us', which compared the crack crisis to 'the struggle for civil rights, the war in Vietnam and the fall of the Nixon presidency'. And two documentaries, CBS's *48 Hours on Crack Street* and NBC's *Cocaine Country* in the summer of 1986, stoked the fire. Crack anxiety reached a fever pitch in the late eighties.

There is no doubt that the effects of crack on poor black neighbourhoods were dire and long-lasting. The media coverage, however, was disproportionately hysterical as well as inaccurate. Journalists were discovered to have invented some particularly lurid crack stories. The so-called phenomenon of crack babies became a national obsession and diverted money away from treatment or prevention. The idea behind the 'crack baby' scare was that women who smoked crack during their pregnancies would give birth to drug-addicted, permanently brain-damaged children and that the crack epidemic, if left unchecked, could result in a whole generation of incapacitated half-wits who would need to be provided for by the state.

Later studies determined that babies born to crack-addicted mothers are underweight and prone to learning difficulties but perfectly capable of growing up normally if given proper care. The real damage is not caused by crack but by being raised by an addict in an unstable, dysfunctional environment.

It is true that crack-related emergency-room admissions jumped precipitously in the mid-eighties. But such figures do not mean the scourge was sweeping the nation. In reality, the average citizen was unaffected by crack, which remained a problem for inner-city blacks. It is only in this context that the word epidemic is appropriate.

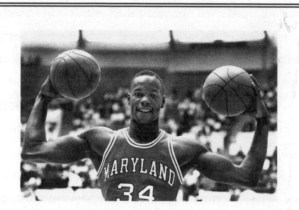

PROFILE: LEN BIAS (1963–86)

At twenty-two years old, Leonard K. Bias, a 6 ft 8 in. basketball star from the University of Maryland, seemed poised for a life of success, riches and women after being drafted by the Boston Celtics, a team that had just won the NBA championships. Only fifty players were signed by the NBA that year, making the odds for the thousands of top college basketball hopefuls slim. But Bias had always stood out from the crowd and everyone – his fans at Northwestern High School, his College Park teammates, politicians in DC who were watching his career with interest – expected nothing less than greatness from this phenomenal young man.

Len was very likeable. He hadn't allowed his godlike status on campus to go to his head; he seemed modest, even goofy. He remained loyal to old friends and relied on the support of his close-knit family. His parents, James, an equipment repair man, and Lonise, a customer service representative at a bank, attended most of his games, providing him and the other students in his dorm with pots of home-cooked stew and spaghetti. They were good, religious people and they wanted their son to be happy and grounded. But it wasn't possible for Len to lead a typical college existence.

Wherever he went, he was showered with adulation and attention. Everyone wanted a piece of him – girls, fans, local newspapers and television channels. Even professors were slightly in awe of him despite his abysmal academic record. Bias had never been an intellectual and with his heavy athletic schedule and active social life he had very little time left for studying. Like many NBA recruits, he was failing most of his classes and probably would not graduate. This didn't really bother Lenny, who was too busy enjoying himself. He liked fast cars as well as glitzy clothes and jewellery – he wore a gold chain with 'BIAS' in diamond letters. He also liked blowing off steam by partying and, as it turned out, taking cocaine.

On 18 June 1986, he sealed the deal with the Celtics and signed an endorsement with Reebok. He was excited and happy but exhausted and overwhelmed by all of the pressure. He needed to unwind. After landing in Washington at about 10 p.m., he dropped his father at home before going back to his dorm. He and his close friend Brian Tribble drove to a liquor store and bought Private Stock Malt Liquor and an $18 bottle of Hennessy. The party began in earnest at 2:30 a.m. when they woke up their roommates Terry Long and David Gregg and removed a large stash of cocaine from its hiding place in a hole in the wall.

The drug scene at the University of Maryland was barely considered a problem by the authorities, who were far more worried about binge drinking. Lenny did not fit the bill of a typical coke user, who was generally thought to be white, artistic and louche. He couldn't be called an addict per se but he had been using cocaine regularly for about eight months, buying a gram at a time from Tribble and generously sharing it with his friends. It is doubtful that Bias, who otherwise treated his body like a temple, sometimes running off calorific beers in the middle of the night, knew much about the substance he was taking. He failed to heed the cardinal rule of seasoned drug users: 'Be mindful of dosage.'

In the dorm Lenny passed around a mirror with a mountain of cocaine which they snorted through red McDonald's straws. They stopped momentarily while Lenny had a heart-to-heart with his old friend Jeff Baxter who disapproved of drug taking. Lenny spoke of the 'crazy life' he was going to lead and how he would need the support of his family. Baxter went to bed at about 3:15 a.m. and the others resumed their binge. 'Don't you think you're overdoing it?' one of them asked Lenny. 'I'm alright,' he said. 'I'm as strong as horse.'

When Bias got up to go to the bathroom, he faltered, sat back and started convulsing. Long, who had taken a course in cardiopulmonary resuscitation, recognised the symptoms of a seizure and wedged the same red McDonald's straws into his mouth in order to prevent him from choking on his own tongue. He then attempted mouth-to-mouth resuscitation while Griggs pinned down Bias's long, twitching legs. At 6:33 a.m. they called the paramedics.

Although Griggs was in a state of shock, he realised that the cocaine needed to be disposed of. With trembling hands he poured the remaining powder into a bag of cookies, spilling half onto the carpet, which he then scrubbed down. Then he woke up Jeff Baxter with the words 'Lenny's in the other room dying.'

When the paramedics examined Bias, they found no activity in his heart. Hauling his cumbersome body onto the stretcher was an awkward affair. Before taking him to the hospital, they asked if he had taken any drugs. 'No,' his friends replied, not wanting to get him into trouble. But Lenny was beyond help. After injecting him with five different drugs, inserting a pacemaker and considering a heart transplant, doctors declared Len Bias dead at 8:55 a.m.

To the 38,000 students at the University of Maryland in 1986, Len Bias's death was comparable to Kennedy's or Lennon's. 'Where were you when Len Bias died?'

was a question they would always be able to answer. His death sent shock waves throughout the college and across the nation and he was given a funeral of almost regal proportions. Over 1,300 people, including the political elite of Maryland, journalists and television crews, filed into the university chapel to gaze on his body in an open casket and hear him eulogised as 'the epitome of the student athlete'.

Jesse Jackson, never one to miss out on a public spectacle, took centre stage at a memorial service for Bias and preached in front of a crowd of 11,000. With his famous flair for rhetoric he likened him to Jesus, Martin Luther King and Gandhi, other martyrs cut short in their prime. Bias was sacrificial victim at the altar of an evil menace to black society: drugs. Drugs, he argued, were more dangerous than the Ku Klux Klan. 'Lenny was vulnerable because all of us are vulnerable. He is being used by God to save a generation,' Jackson concluded. Mrs Bias told the crowd that her son's last words to her had been 'love you, Mom'.

On 24 June, the state medical examiner officially announced that Bias had died of 'cocaine intoxication'. He had taken 5 grams of cocaine, more than three times a fatal dose. Another 8 grams had been found in the cookie bag.

When dealers found out that the cocaine had been 89 per cent pure – twice as strong as most cocaine on the street – they started referring to their own product as 'Len Bias' to denote quality and boost sales.

THE IDOL DEFILED

Members of the US Congress, along with the rest of the country, were dismayed by the unfolding story of Bias's drug-induced demise. They had watched him on television and in the sports pages of the *Washington Post*. To them, he was the athlete next door, with a place in their hearts.

On the date of his overdose Bias possessed an invitation to lunch on Capitol Hill. House Speaker Tip O'Neill and Senator Ted Kennedy had asked coach Red Auerbach to bring him. Now he was disgraced and their cherished Celtics blemished by scandal.

Bias had been expected to rewrite the NBA record books. Instead he found his place in forensic history – he became a standard against which fatal overdoses would be measured and compared.

ANTI-DRUG ABUSE ACT OF 1986

Len Bias's death coincided with the crack scare and even though what killed him was powder, his overdose was none-theless associated with crack. The tragedy cued the passage of the most important anti-drug bill to date.

During the summer of 1986, a Senate subcommittee met to discuss the escalating crack problem. Bias's name featured eleven times. The resulting recommendations were turned into law with the Anti-Drug Abuse Act of October 1986. This law was rushed through speedily, and some say carelessly, due to the belief that emergency measures were required to deal with the crisis.

The act, which was followed by the Anti-Drug Abuse Act of 1988, was Reagan's first major piece of legislation in his War on Drugs. Over $1.6 billion was devoted to the cause, with $575 million going towards catching smugglers and $250 million towards education. The bill made bail and parole more difficult, and brought in mandatory minimum sentencing for drug offences, including the notorious 100-to-1 sentencing disparity between powdered and crack cocaine. The possession of only 5 grams of crack (about five tablespoons) led to a minimum sentence of five years whereas you had to possess 500 grams (the amount a trafficker might be carrying) of powdered cocaine to receive the same sentence.

Congress, which had been greatly influenced by the firestorm around Len Bias's death, made a judgement call on the relative evils of powdered cocaine and crack, deeming the latter far more dangerous. Without much evidence, they deduced that crack users were more likely to commit crimes and that the drug led to psychosis.

LET THE PUNISHMENT FIT THE CRIME

Because cocaine and crack users divided along racial lines, the sentencing disparity between the two led to the disproportionate imprisonment of young black men. It is for this reason that the Anti-Drug Abuse Acts of 1986 and 1988 are held responsible by the left for a lost generation of black men, locked away for minor offences for years on end and ill equipped to deal with the world when released

By 1989 a high percentage of criminal court cases were for drug offences. Most arrests were of low-level users and dealers rather than of high-level suppliers, a problem that still exists today. The legislation did not, therefore, clamp down on the kingpins or traffickers and instead upped the ante on the punitive turn that started with Nixon and resulted in the swelling of America's prison population, which grew fivefold in thirty years.

The anti-drug acts contributed to America's expanding prison population – American prisons are bursting at the seams and cannot be built quickly enough. In 1980 there were fewer than 500,000 prisoners in the US; by 2012 there were over 1.6 million. This is the highest incarceration rate in the world, with roughly 743 inmates per 300,000 people, beating countries like Russia, Iran and China. Another way of looking at this is that America has 5 per cent of the world's population and 25 per cent of its prisoners.

PROFILE: WHITNEY HOUSTON (1963–2012)

Whitney Houston is one of the most lauded female singers of all time and the most influential pop diva of them all. Whitney had 'the voice' of her generation, the voice that is said to send shivers down one's spine and inspire feelings of almost religious transcendence. Her beautiful mezzo-soprano was a technical tour de force with incredible range and depth that was, nevertheless, pure and light, even angelic. Critics, grasping for verbal definition, have described its 'velvety depths', 'ringing and airy heights' its 'shimmering melismas' and the fact that it is an 'aspirational' and 'hopeful' voice.

Aspirational is a loaded but apt word for Whitney Houston, who, perhaps thanks to the guiding hand of Clive Davis, her Svengali at Arista Records, appealed to both black and white audiences alike. It helped that she was stunningly beautiful with high cheekbones, a huge winning smile and legs that went on for miles. She had already had a successful career as a teenage model and was one of the first black models to grace the cover of *Seventeen* magazine.

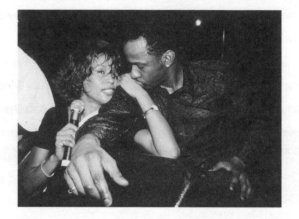

Whitney didn't need technical gimmicks or showmanship like Madonna or Michael Jackson and instead just stood on stage in her sparking, elegant gowns and delivered exquisite live performances. She appeared untouchable and slightly aloof but never bratty or difficult. This air of mystery was maintained in part because she rarely gave interviews.

Some grumbled that Whitney was too sugar-coated and that her urban pop confections lacked depth or soul. In other words, she wasn't black enough. Still, the hits kept coming and her upbeat music videos were played repeatedly on MTV, a predominantly white channel.

Most of Whitney's fame was based on music produced

during the seven years prior to her 30th birthday, between the release of her first album, *Whitney Houston*, in 1985 and her starring role in *The Bodyguard* in 1992. In 1987, at the age of twenty-four, Forbes ranked her as one of the top ten entertainers in the world with a fortune of $44 million. By 1988, she had beaten the Beatles' record with seven consecutive No. 1 Billboard Hot 100 hits and had a collection of prestigious awards including multiple Grammys.

Whitney was an American treasure, feted by Presidents and statesmen and friends with Nelson Mandela. There were, however, small chinks in the armour already, which many blame on her union with Bobby Brown, a singer five years her junior with an established criminal past. When Whitney clapped eyes on him at the 1989 Soul Train Music Awards – a black awards ceremony where she was booed for being an 'Oreo' (black on the outside, white on the inside) – she said to herself, 'This man is going to be my husband.' Bobby would do much to infuse Whitney's whitewashed image with a strong dose of ghetto street cred. He also stopped those niggling lesbian rumours.

Whitney and Bobby had entered into one of those classically toxic domestic partnerships, à la Ike and Tina, an abusive but passionate 'can't live with or without you' scenario. There is no doubt that Whitney loved Bobby. She may even have been grateful to him for destroying that irritating princess reputation of hers. She didn't like being thought of as prissy and told *Rolling Stone* magazine that she could 'get down, really freakin' dirty'. Like Katharine Hepburn in *The Philadelphia Story*, she wanted to be taken off her pedestal. She eventually got her wish but Bobby was always blamed for it.

The nineties was a decade of decline. In 1994, she was two hours late to a White House dinner where she was supposed to perform for Nelson Mandela. By 1996, she was taking drugs every day. It all started 'getting heavy' after *The Bodyguard*, she told Oprah. Bobby taught her how to lace cocaine into marijuana to even out the drugs, 'kind of like speed-balling where you mix cocaine and heroin', she helpfully explained. Oprah nodded politely.

In 1999 Whitney attempted a comeback but was forced to cancel five concerts. Her was voice was ruined by cigarettes and drugs. Pictures of her looking emaciated and sick emerged in tabloids, some of which erroneously reported that she had died from an overdose.

Several well-documented episodes, like Whitney's 2002 'crack is whack' interview with Diane Sawyer, helped shatter her image. With a raspy, broken voice and an arrogant but deranged manner, Whitney broke into a rage when asked about crack. 'First of all. Let's get one thing straight. Crack is cheap. I make way too much money to ever smoke crack ... Okay? We don't do crack. We don't do that. Crack is whack,' she said. That same year, she was sued for $100 million by her father's business partner, Kevin Skinner. The suit was later dropped. Many of her dodgy associates wanted to cash in on the Whitney gravy train, especially now that she was vulnerable.

Whitney's private chauffeur Al Bowman spoke to the *Daily Mirror* about his famous client after her death, saying that she was the worst-behaved star he had ever worked for. Whitney's raging drug habit took them into the heart of the ghetto as she sought out crack dealers. She had no compunction about smoking crack in the backseat of the limo while seated next to her six-year-old daughter, Bobbi Kristina. 'Baby, Mommy and Daddy are doing adult things,' she would tell her. Bowman's revelations did not come as much of a surprise as Whitney had already made the mistake of appearing in her husband's infamous 2005 reality television show *Being Bobby Brown*, filmed the year before their divorce. According to Mark Seal in *Vanity Fair*, 'Whitney gradually descends into a chain-smoking, apple martini-drinking, foulmouthed, wild-haired shrew' who yells 'kiss my ass' and 'hell to the no'.

Bobby Brown doesn't fare much better – he rubs Preparation H haemorrhoid cream under his eyes to prevent bags and warns his millionaire children not to shoplift. Bobby maintains that the show revealed Whitney's true self, that her saintly image was bullshit. Others in Whitney's inner circle say that she was a good Christian, a loving mother and a vibrant and spirited soul who couldn't conquer her demons. Whitney Houston's faith in Jesus Christ remained strong through her highs and lows. She prayed to God to help her make a comeback, hiring a voice coach and going into rehab. She wanted a facelift but was turned down by doctors because of her bad heart, which was damaged by years of cocaine abuse.

Clive Davis believed that Whitney was ready for her second act. She had fared tolerably well – with

only some booing from the Australians – during her
2010 'Nothing but Love' tour and she had just finished
filming and recording a soundtrack for her new film,
Sparkle. On set she was drug-free and professional.
Clive Davis invited her to perform at a pre-Grammy
party in February and Whitney turned up in Los
Angeles a few days early with her new, much younger
lover, Ray J, in tow. This part-time singer and reality TV
actor is most famous for leaking Kim Kardashian's 2007
sex tape.

Whitney spent her last twenty-four hours alone. An
assistant came to get her ready for the pre-Grammy party
and found her face down in a foot of warm bathwater
with blood pouring out her nose. She was pronounced
dead at the scene. The cause of Whitney Houston's death
was accidental drowning caused by heart disease and
cocaine use. The coroner's report described a woman of
healthy weight with a perforated septum and scald burns
and cuts on her upper lip and body. Powdered cocaine
was found in her room along with prescription medica-
tions and marijuana. On her bathroom counter there
was a 'small spoon with a white crystal-like substance in
it', a polite description for crack.

Celebrity guests including Tom Hanks, Neil Young
and P Diddy, who were now streaming into the lobby
of the Beverly Hilton Hotel to hear Whitney sing, were
instead greeted with the shocking news of the 48-year-
old legend's death. Her comeback had turned into her
wake and her story could no longer have a fairy-tale
ending. Drugs had stolen her voice, health, looks and

dignity together with her $100 million fortune. The career of one of the greatest singers in the world had gone down in twelve inches of blood-tinted water in the bottom of the bath.

CRACK NO MORE

Violent crimes increased in the second half of the twentieth century, with homicide rates in the US doubling between the 1960s and the 1990s. Between 1984 and 1989, violent crimes increased by 5 per cent, and would, according to statisticians, keep on rising. But then in the late nineties, the reverse happened: crime dropped and homicide rates dipped back to early 1960s levels. In *Freakonomics*, Steven Levitt and Stephen J. Dubner attribute this to legalisation of abortion in the seventies (which reduced the number of future criminals being born). Another explanation is that the reduction in crime was partly related to the containment of the crack problem.

Crack does not cause crime, but the need to acquire it does. A 2005 study conducted by the National Bureau of Economic Research found that, between 1984 and 1994, murder rates for young black men nearly doubled, foetal death rates and weapons arrests in poor black neighbourhoods rose by 25 per cent and the number of children in foster care doubled. The same was not true for whites. The study claims that crack was directly responsible for the spike in figures.

Crack rates climbed precipitously in 1985, peaked in 1989 and dropped steadily in the 1990s. By 2000 most of the awful social consequences of crack had disappeared and there was no longer a link between crack and violence. Few new users were recruited and existing users were ageing addicts without much energy for crime.

THE END OF THE AFFAIR

The decline of crack was part of the overall decline in American cocaine usage that started in the mid-to-late eighties and continued (but at a slower rate) during the new millennium. In 1982 there were 10.5 million cocaine users in the US and by 2008 only 5.3 million. According to the US government (which may exaggerate figures for the sake of their argument), the value of the US cocaine market fell even more precipitously, from $134 billion in 1982 to $35 billion in 2008, because of cheaper prices and reduced purity.

The end of America's affair with cocaine can be attributed to several factors, including supply reduction through coca eradication polices in Colombia. The media scare and stigma associated with crack undoubtedly had an effect on the young, who decided to steer clear of cocaine. Tastes change, drugs go in and out of fashion and cocaine no longer reflected the zeitgeist. Today's young Americans can hardly be called abstemious. They have just switched vices, favouring easily procured prescription drugs such as Adderall and, to a lesser extent, crystal meth.

5

GLOBAL SPILL: PRODUCING AND SMUGGLING

MEXICO

BEYOND THE PALE

On 23 March 2013, seven corpses were ceremoniously arranged in a row of white chairs in the town centre of Uruapan, a city in the Mexican state of Michoacán. Their hands and feet were bound and ominous messages were attached to their chests with ice picks. Today, these types of murders are the norm in Mexico, a part of daily life. There have been over 60,000 drug-related deaths in Mexico since 2006. The population is so hardened to violence that only truly gruesome acts such as the hanging of severed heads from freeway overpasses and the sewing of human faces onto footballs are reported by the national media. International papers have focused on a few compelling stories such as the *feminicidio* (feminicide) or targeted killing of women in Ciudad Juárez. The gunning-down of Maria Santos Gorrostieta, a 36-year-old mother and former small-town mayor also made headlines.

Mexican *narcos* (drug lords) have a macabre sense of humour and flair for the theatrical. They have responded well to the internet age. Snuff videos are put on YouTube and *narcomensajes* (drug messages) are posted online or scrolled on corpses and hung from banners. Victims are tortured in cruel and unusual ways designed to maximise suffering; hands are severed so that victims bleed to death slowly, or bones are scraped with ice-picks. Sometimes, the punishment will match the so-called crime and a spy will have his eyes gouged out, a tattletale will have his lips chopped off, a pig's head will be stuck on the body of someone who was greedy, and so on.

Becoming a cold-blooded killer takes some getting used to. Novices must lose their inhibitions about death and learn to treat people like slabs of meat. That is why one cartel, *La Familia*, likes to employ butchers and men who work in taco joints. A member described the process by which new recruits are inured to the violence of their job: 'This is how we put them to the test. We made them kill. Then we made them quarter the bodies, because the new people coming in lose their fear by cutting off an arm or a leg or something.' Some employees are desensitised from the outset. *El Pozolero,* or the stew-maker, from the outskirts of Tijuana had no compunction about dissolving 300 bodies in acid in 2009. He was paid a handsome $600 a week for his troubles.

The majority of drug murders in Mexico are committed by stealth assassins who use hit-and-run tactics that are very difficult to police. The bodies may be dumped on roadsides, thrown in shallow graves or dissolved in acid. Between 2005 and 2010, kidnappings rose by 317 per cent and, since 2006, beheadings have become commonplace. It is thought that the cartels got their inspiration from the *Kaibiles*, Guatemalan mercenaries who took to decapitation during their long civil war. A famous incident in 2006, when *La Familia* rolled five severed heads across the floor of a disco in Michoacán, did much to popularise the phenomenon.

THE DRUG MARKET

The American drug market is worth $60 billion a year, about half of which goes directly to the Mexican drug cartels. While $30 billion is only 3 per cent of Mexico's $1.16 trillion GDP, it is enough to corrupt institutions and provide indirect employment to hundreds of thousands of people. Drug trafficking is the second largest source of revenue after oil, beating out remittances and tourism.

About 90 per cent of the cocaine smuggled into the US is transported through Mexico – the rest comes through the Caribbean. Even though the cocaine market is about half what it was in the late eighties, the great mark-up from leaf to street sale – a kilogram sells for $2,200 in the jungle and $27,000 wholesale in the US – makes it well worth their efforts. It is estimated that 34 per cent of the cartels' revenue comes from cocaine (the percentage would be much larger were it not for the Colombian suppliers), with heroin, marijuana and crystal meth each providing 17 per cent and the rest coming from non-drug sources like extortion. While cocaine is not the only source of income for the cartels, its contribution is significant.

THE BACKSTORY

Sinaloa is part of the Golden Triangle, the historic drug-producing heartland of Mexico that also includes Durango and Chihuahua. Sinaloa has been the epicentre of smuggling since the Mexican War of Independence (1810–21), when Sinaloans dealt in contraband silver and weaponry. During the late nineteenth century, Chinese immigrants grew opium in the region and in the 1960s the West's sudden appetite for marijuana – the Mexican variety was named 'Acapulco Gold' – turned small-time Sinaloan hustlers into rich drug lords.

When President Reagan and VP George Bush started policing the Florida coastline in 1982, the cocaine industry was hit hard. Instead of fighting the American military apparatus head-on, the Colombian traffickers decided to enlist the help of the Sinaloans, whose well-established marijuana and heroin smuggling routes through the longer US–Mexican border could also be used to transport cocaine.

The Mexicans started off as distributors who collected a fee for delivering Colombian cocaine. But in the late eighties, when America put pressure on Colombia through asset seizure and extradition, the Colombians got worried and ceded more control to the Mexican traffickers. Slowly but surely the Mexicans gained the upper hand, first demanding payment in cocaine rather than money, and then taking over from the Colombians entirely after Pablo Escobar's death in 1993, when they became the most powerful drug traffickers in the world.

In the 1980s Mexican drug trafficking was run by the Guadalajara cartel with Miguel Ángel Félix Gallardo, a Sinaloan known as 'The Godfather' or 'the Boss of Bosses', at the helm. Gallardo got overly confident and ordered the kidnapping and killing of DEA agent Enrique (Kiki) Camarena. In response to US pressure, the Mexican government, which was still more powerful than the traffickers, had the 43-year-old arrested and imprisoned in April of 1989. From prison, Gallardo oversaw his drug dominions and organised a *narco* summit in the resort town of Acapulco to discuss decentralisation.

The Acapulco summit divvied up Gallardo's empire into discrete trafficking plazas, which controlled the flow of goods, usually drugs, in and out of their territory and unintentionally created the current situation of competing cartels. The breakup of the Guadalajara cartel led to increased violence during the 1990s. The violence, however, was caused by inter-cartel warfare and ordinary citizens were mostly left alone. This all changed in the new millennium and coincided with the transition from dictatorship to democracy.

DICTATORSHIP AND DEMOCRACY

For seventy-one years (1929–2000) Mexico was run by the Institutional Revolutionary Party (PRI), oxymoronic since a party is rarely both institutional and revolutionary. Corruption was an instrumental part of the PRI's stifling success and everyone (from the police to the military to governmental officials) knew their place in the hierarchy of bribes.

Drug trafficking was unofficially condoned by the PRI as long the government received its cut. Government corruption was so endemic that President Salinas's brother, Raúl, is thought to have overseen drug shipments out of

Mexico. It is President Salinas (whose presidency ran from 1988 to 1994) who helped Bill Clinton push through the North Atlantic Free Trade Agreement (NAFTA) in 1994. NAFTA, which lifted trade barriers between the US, Canada and Mexico and made it easier for goods to cross the border, proved a boon to traffickers by quadrupling the inter-border traffic.

In 2000, the PRI reign came to an end with the historic election of Vicente Fox of the right-of-centre National Action Party (PAN). Fox, a rich Coca-Cola executive with a cowboy style, was a weak character who excelled at entertaining dignitaries but was not up to the monumental task of filling the power vacuum left by the PRI. Their corrupt 'arrangement' with the drug cartels had, to a certain extent, kept the violence under control. Without it, all hell broke loose.

The Mexican drug war began in earnest in the autumn of 2004. The first outbreak occurred in Nuevo Laredo, a border city directly across from Dallas which is one of the main export hubs for both legal and illegal goods into the US. The bloodshed continued through the summer of 2005 and began spreading to other parts of Mexico. When Felipe Calderón, a Harvard-educated lawyer (also of the PAN party), ran for President, he campaigned on the promise of solving the drug crisis. Within ten days of assuming office on 1 December 2006, he declared war on the drug lords and immediately sent troops into Michoacán. During the next few years he enlisted over 50,000 federal soldiers and policemen to go after the drug cartels.

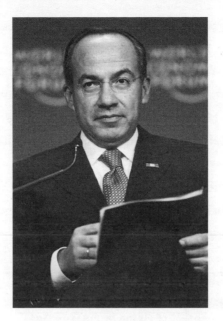

Felipe Calderón

The drug war only worsened, getting particularly bad in 2008. In 2009, Ciudad Juárez received the dubious honour of most dangerous city in the world outside of a war zone, with 193 murders per 100,000 people. In 2010, there were 15,000 drug-related murders in Mexico and another 16,000 in 2011. By 2012, the Mexican people were fed up and voted the PRI back into power. Many hope that the old imperfect order will be restored, even if it means cutting a deal with the cartels. But after twelve years of lawlessness, it will be difficult to return to status quo.

CARTELS

Since the 2000s, eight drug cartels have terrorised Mexico: the Sinaloa cartel; the Gulf cartel; the *Zetas* (originally part of Gulf); the Tijuana cartel, aka the Arellano-Félix Organization (AFO); the Juárez cartel; *La Familia* (now disbanded); the Knights Templar (originally part of *La Familia*) and the Beltrán Leyva cartel (originally part of Sinaloa). Currently, the Sinaloans and the *Zetas* are the pre-eminent cartels, battling with each other and the military for control of Mexico. Broadly speaking, the Sinaloans dominate the west of Mexico (sixteen states), the *Zetas* dominate the east (seventeen states) and they both make incursions into the other's territory.

PROFILE: EL CHAPO DE SINALOA (1954—)

'Chapo' Guzmán, the most wanted drug trafficker in the world and the head of the Sinaloa cartel, has eluded the law for decades. He has outlived Pablo Escobar, who died at forty-five, by over a decade and has surpassed the Colombian in terms of influence. In 2009, Forbes magazine got into trouble for putting Chapo on their list of billionaires. A few months later, he ranked 41st in their list of influential people for his role in overseeing 'anywhere from $6 billion to $19 billion in cocaine shipments to the US over the past eight years'.

Joaquín Guzmán Loera – later dubbed 'Chapo' or 'Shorty'; he's 5 ft 6 in. – was born on Christmas Day in 1954 in La Tuna, an impoverished town of about 200 people, at the base of the Sierra Madre mountains in Sinaloa. The area is still terribly poor – it costs a mere

$35 to have someone murdered – and Chapo's childhood was suitably miserable. During the day he toiled in the fields and at night he was beaten. His father, who was ostensibly a cattle rancher, was actually a *gomero*, or an opium grower, with connections to the Sinaloa drug trade. This is how Chapo got started.

As a teenager, Chapo delivered drugs from his home town to bigger cities, exhibiting a steeliness that caught the attention of his superiors. If a shipment went missing or got lost, he never raised his voice or lost his cool. Instead, he calmly shot the culprit in the head. By the early eighties, Gallardo, the 'Godfather' of the Guadalajara cartel, put Chapo in charge of coordinating flights of cocaine from Colombia to Mexico. When the Guadalajara cartel broke up in 1989, Chapo was chosen to run the important Sinaloa plaza and went about transforming it into the pre-eminent cartel that it is today by dominating the cocaine trade.

Chapo may have as many as 150,000 workers, but fewer than 150 of them are official employees. Cocaine is an expensive drug because of the risks involved for transporters and because thousands of people – from 'falcons' or citizen spies to taxi drivers – need to be paid off along the way. Keeping so many people under control is not easy but Chapo possesses the right combination of charm and authority. His small stature, nasal voice and very casual dress sense (like Escobar, he favours jeans, baseball caps and trainers) endear him to the common man. Everyone is taken in by his pleasant and affable manner when they meet him and quickly forget about the thousands of people he has quietly executed.

A psychological assessment of Chapo conducted while he was in prison concluded that 'revenge is not something he exacts with the immediacy of an impulsive person'. Chapo never forgets an enemy but he is patient, calculating and willing to hold back in order to exact the most appropriate punishment. Even though he is illiterate, he keeps tabs on his complex business with detailed account books that have now all been digitalised.

Chapo is very inventive and has tested all sorts of methods for hiding cocaine, once buying a cannery so that he could stuff red chillies with the drug. He has inserted cocaine into fire extinguishers, candy bars, baby dolls, fish, sharks, FedEx parcels and statues of Jesus and the Virgin Mary. Other cartels copy his techniques and now factories in Mexico build cars with secret cocaine compartments that can only be opened by setting them on fire.

Chapo is an expert on transportation. He flies cocaine in 747 airliners or moves it in chartered cruise ships. He oversees the construction of semi-submersible submarines built in the Amazon at $2 million apiece. Because only eighteen inches are visible above water, they are very difficult to spot. If discovered, they are flooded and sink to the bottom of the ocean without a trace other than the crew bobbing at the surface in life jackets. A 32-foot semi-submersible carrying 5.8 tons was discovered near the coast of Oaxaca in July of 2008. Chapo will always be remembered for the underground tunnels between Mexico and the US that he built during the late eighties and early nineties.

In May 1990, customs agents in Douglas, Arizona broke into a warehouse and uncovered a 270-foot, concrete-lined and air-conditioned passageway that led to a false floor under a pool table in a house in Mexico. The floor could be raised by activating the garden hose and the drugs were lowered onto carts with pulleys. Chapo was pleased with the results and praised the architect for building him 'a fucking cool tunnel'.

Another even more impressive tunnel from Tijuana to California was discovered a few years later. This one was 65 ft deep and 1,452 ft long. Chapo's tunnels allowed him to move multiple tons of cocaine across the border each month. In order to keep costs down, he rounded up migrant workers and executed them once their work was done – he couldn't risk them squealing.

In 1993, Chapo was arrested and sentenced to twenty years in prison. In 1995, he was transferred to Puente Grande, a maximum-security prison where it didn't take long for him to get the entire staff on side. Those who resisted were shown a list with their family members' names and addresses. They all chose to spare their loved ones and cooperate.

Chapo oversaw his business from prison but also found time for fun. He wandered around unaccompanied and was fed delicious meals by his personal chef. He brought in mariachi bands, alcohol and prostitutes from the outside world and threw parties for the inmates. During one Christmas Eve celebration, he and his guests dined on lobster soup, filet mignon and whisky. Chapo also liked playing chess, basketball and volleyball – he is very competitive. Sometimes, he would watch Disney films with fellow inmates and eat popcorn and ice cream.

Chapo is a romantic at heart. He has several wives who, as the mothers of his sons, are very important to him. In prison, he met 27-year-old Zulema Yulia Hernández, the greatest love of his life. Zulema, also from Sinaloa, was a former policewoman who had switched sides and become a *narco*. She was tall and fair skinned with caramel-coloured hair and 'a near perfect body' according to the inmates. The two fell passionately in love and he dictated touching letters to her with lines like 'I send you a kiss of honey and a hug that makes you shake with emotion'. Chapo arranged for Zulema to be transferred out of prison. She was later murdered by the *Zetas*.

When the Mexican government approved a law that made it easier to extradite criminals to the United States, Chapo decided that it was time to leave prison – nobody knows why he chose to stay in prison for as long as he did. It cost him $2.5 million to bribe the right people and in January 2001, he was smuggled out of Puente Grande in a laundry cart. Henceforth, the prison would be jokingly referred to as Puerta Grande, or 'large door'.

Chapo's comical prison escape coincided with the end of PRI rule and the beginning of the drug war. Even Chapo was not immune to the violence and he suffered a series of blows towards the end of 2004. First, his brother was murdered. Then his son Ivan Archivaldo or 'Chapito' (Little Chapo) was arrested but eventually acquitted for money laundering. Chapito's arrest showed that the children of traffickers, known as *narco* juniors, were now being targeted by the law. In 2008, his other son, Edgar Guzman López, a typical *narco* junior, was murdered. He was twenty-two years old.

Narco juniors are a new, sanitised breed of drug trafficker. They are shielded from the family business during their rich, gilded childhoods and teenage years and only introduced to the trade, usually by running a front business, in their twenties. They attend fancy private schools and foreign universities where they study business or economics and learn several languages. They do not wear the garish *narco* outfits of their fathers, preferring a sleek, metropolitan look.

The *Zetas* have been poaching some of Chapo's business in recent years. The Sinaloa cartel still controls 40–60 per cent of the Mexican cocaine trade but they are now on the defensive. Chapo is increasingly isolated, rarely straying from his trusted mountainous retreat. But his occasional appearances are legendary. In 2005, for example, he graced a medium-sized restaurant in Nuevo Laredo with his presence. A group of bodyguards entered first and warned the diners of what was about to happen. All mobiles would be confiscated and nobody could leave, but they didn't need to fear for their lives. Chapo was true to his word. He took a seat in the back and enjoyed a large meal of Sinaloan shrimp and beef for a few hours. Everyone's meals were paid for.

In November 2006, Emma Coronel, seventeen-year-old niece of Nacho Coronel, a famous trafficker known as the 'Crystal King', organised a dance in her bid to win a beauty pageant and become Queen of Canelas. The night of the dance, 200 bodyguards drove into the town on motorbikes and barricaded the street leading up to the dance hall. Six planes then landed. One of them carried the group Los Canelos de Durango, another carried Nacho Coronel and a third carried Chapo Guzmán. A few months later, on her 18th birthday, Emma Coronel became Chapo's fourth wife. It is very difficult to refuse a trafficker's marriage proposal. In 2011 Emma gave birth in an LA county hospital – she is a US citizen – and snuck back over the border with Chapo's twin daughters.

The government receives countless tips about Chapo's whereabouts but most of them are false leads. Will Chapo ever be caught? Or will he, with the help of his devoted followers, escape detection forever? *Narco* singers have faith in their favourite outlaw. And anonymous *narco* messages scrolled on banners concur. 'You'll never find El Chapo. Not the priests, not the government.'

PROFILE: THE *ZETAS*

The Gulf cartel, which is based in the north-eastern state of Tamaulipas, is one of the oldest crime syndicates in Mexico. In 1997, Osiel Cárdenas Guillén, a former car thief with the moniker of '*El Mata Amigos*', or 'The Friend Killer', murdered his way to the top of the cartel. He then had the inspired idea of creating an enforcement wing to defend the cartel against its numerous enemies, a decision the Gulf cartel would come to regret.

Osiel Cárdenas sought skilled recruits, so he turned to the Mexican army for help. He persuaded Arturo Guzmán Decena to defect from the Special Forces Airmobile Group (GAFE), an elite internationally trained corps with the motto *Todo por México* (Everything for Mexico). Arturo Guzmán Decena, who had originally been sent to Taumaulipas to fight the drug cartels, switched sides and brought forty of his army colleagues along with him. They named themselves the *Zetas* after a GAFE radio signal. Guzmán was reborn as Z-1 and the leaders that followed him were named Z-2, Z-3 etc.

The *Zetas* are notorious for their unnecessary savagery and total disregard for human life. They took drug violence to a whole new level with their penchant for kidnappings, beheadings, extortion, torture and violent exhibitionism, tactics that would soon be copied by other cartels. They also developed new operational strategies, making use of

semi-autonomous cells which retain their independence
so long as they send money back to the *Zetas*.

The *Zetas* began to outclass their Gulf mentors in
the art of coercion, domination and territorial expansion. When the *Zetas* and Gulf split in February 2010,
violence erupted all over the north-east of Mexico.
While the Gulf cartel is a shadow of its former self, the
Zetas have gone from strength to strength. They have
significantly expanded their north-eastern base and
have a very strong presence in Guatemala, a country
that provides them with mercenaries and heavy-grade
weaponry and is useful as a cocaine supply route and
shipping point.

Immigration to the United States has dropped in recent
years, mostly because of the economic recession but
partly out of fear of the *Zetas*. The *Zetas* will kidnap just
about anybody, with the knowledge that even impoverished people have relations who care about them. So they
abduct busloads of Central American migrants on route
to the US and take them to ranches and torture them
until their families transfer small sums of money to the
Zetas via Western Union. In the infamous San Fernando
massacre of August 2010, seventy-two migrants were
summarily executed for no apparent reason.

The scope of the *Zetas'* ambitions is large. They
are not content to limit themselves to drug trafficking, which now accounts for only 20 per cent of their
revenue. They rule Nuevo Laredo with an iron fist,
totally silencing the media and extorting every business in sight, and they hope to do the same in the rest of

Mexico. They are also trying to emerge as a global force, with tentacles spreading into Africa and Europe.

NARCO CULTURE

Amongst the poor there is a surprising degree of sympathy for the drug-traffickers, who are sometimes referred to as *los valientes,* or the brave ones, especially in the north where the drug war rages. Small boys dream of becoming *narcos* and there is vibrant drug culture, or *narcocultura,* with its own music, religion and fashion.

Narcocorridos are ballads that recount the exploits of famous drug traffickers. Los Tigres del Norte wrote the first *narcocorrido* in 1974 and the genre is still thriving. Traffickers enjoy the notoriety of being sung about and will commission a musician to write a song about them, pay for a recording session and then invite him to perform the song live at a *narco* party.

Drug barons tend to the neo-classical in the design of their mansions. They like columns and lofty interiors, compounded by the glitzy and ornamental. Restrained good taste is not the aim.

Despite their sinful lives, *narcos* are interested in looking after themselves in perpetuity. Their family members build them marble and jewel-encrusted mausoleums (sometimes air-conditioned) that can cost $100,000, and bury them in *narco* cemeteries – the most famous, Jardines del Humaya, is in Culiacán. The *narcos* lie in luxury coffins with mobile phones to hand in the event of resurrection.

Criminals rarely condemn themselves to hell and Mexican drug traffickers are no exception. They justify their behaviour through their own *narco* religion, which is an amalgamation of Catholicism, indigenous culture and, in the case of *'El Más Loco'*, former leader of the *La Familia* cartel, evangelical Christianity. He wrote a bible of sorts called *Pensamientos*, or Thoughts, with helpful aphorisms for his disciples such as: 'Don't view obstacles as problems but accept them and discover in them the opportunity to improve yourself.'

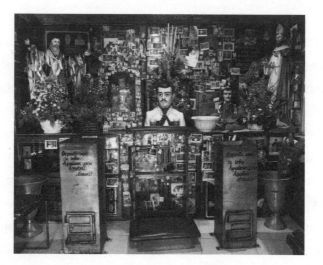

Shrine to Jesús Malverde

Two so-called saints figure prominently in *narco* religion, Jesús Malverde and Santa Muerte. Jesús Malverde was a late-nineteenth-century Sinaloan bandit who, like Robin Hood, stole from the rich to feed the poor and is greatly admired by drug traffickers, who flock to his shrine in Sinaloa. Malverde has short hair, a thick moustache and always wears a black tie or scarf around his neck. Santa Muerte or Holy Death is a grim reaper-like figure with hollowed eyes and a scythe. Neither Malverde nor Santa Muerte is officially sanctioned by the Catholic Church, although many rural churches end up accepting generous donations from traffickers referred to as *narco limosnas* or *narco* alms.

MONEY LAUNDERING

Drugs usually get sold for cash, which either gets shipped back to Mexico, a rather cumbersome affair, or deposited into American banks, a very risky affair. In either case, there is a lot of illegal money floating around that needs to be dealt with. Sticking it under the floorboards is one option and investing it is another. In June 2012 it was discovered that the brother of the second highest-up *Zeta* leader was backing an American horse racing racket called Tremor Enterprises.

We live in an age that accommodates launderers. In 1979 there were only about seventy banks in offshore tax havens while today there are thousands. New York and London are now the money laundering capitals of the world. During the global financial meltdown a good deal was struck between banks which were having trouble finding liquid funds and criminals who needed to house their hot money.

There have been several high-profile cases of money laundering in recent years. The business news website Bloomberg reported that between 2003 and 2008 (the height of the drug war), Wachovia, which was bought out by Wells Fargo, allowed Mexican drug cartels to launder $110 million. They also failed to notice over $400 billion worth of transactions using '*casas de cambios*' or exchange houses. Wells Fargo had to pay a hefty sum after it was discovered that planes loaded with tens of thousands of kilos of cocaine had been purchased with Wachovia money.

In 2012, British bank HSBC paid $1.9 billion – the largest penalty in US banking history – for multiple charges including laundering $881 million for Mexican and Colombian drug cartels. Their CEO expressed little remorse and the bank was able to pay the fine, the equivalent of one month's profits, with relative ease. Even though harsher restrictions are being placed on banks, who promise to be more careful about where their money comes from, it is likely that many instances of laundering will still go undetected.

How many businesses are bought with the spoils of a dirty war? To what degree is Mexico's legal economy propped up by the flow of illegal goods? And how many international banks are happy to invest money earned through extortion and torture? Some argue that until there is a globalised effort to stop the flow of illegal money, there is no point in spraying coca and seizing loads of cocaine.

ALL GUNS BLAZING

Guns are difficult to procure in Mexico because of the country's strict laws. But because America's gun laws are wonderfully lax, cartels pay 'straw buyers' a few hundred dollars to legally purchase guns in Texas, California, Arizona and New Mexico. These states uphold the second amendment to such a degree that there are over 6,700 gun stores within a few hours' drive of the border.

The majority (90 per cent according to some surveys) of guns confiscated from the cartels have been traced back to America through their serial numbers. This so-called Mexican trampoline whereby drugs are smuggled into the US and weapons are brought back (often in the same vehicle) is possible because of the volume of border traffic, with thousands of trucks passing through each day. Only a small percentage of these can be checked by the border patrol.

Even though 30,000 Americans die from guns each year, the National Rifle Association's grip on American legislation is too strong to be broken by any mere President. Obama hasn't even been able to reinstate the ban on semi-automatic weapons that lapsed under George W. Bush in 2004, the very year that the drug war in Mexico took off. While the Obama administration has at least acknowledged 'co-responsibility' in the problem of arms trafficking, most Americans will remain indifferent to the plight of Mexico until the drug violence begins affecting them directly.

So far, despite some notable exceptions, America has been mostly untouched by Mexico's troubles. In Arizona, crime actually fell by 35 per cent between 2004 and 2008. And in 2010, there were only five murders in El Paso, Texas, which is just across from Ciudad Juárez, one of the deadliest cities in Mexico. This is surprising given the strong cultural and familial cross-border ties but is partly explained by the fact that drug dealing in America is not centrally controlled by the cartels as it is in Mexico.

Another explanation is that America has a functioning state and Mexico does not. Americans perhaps justifiably point out that they cannot be blamed for a corrupt, inefficient country where policemen are bribed and journalists gunned down for publishing unpleasant articles. This may be so, but it's also true that America buys Mexican drugs, launders Mexican drug money and provides Mexico with lethal weapons. Drug production and consumption is a collaborative effort and all parties should accept equal responsibility.

PRODUCING AND SMUGGLING
WHO DOES WHAT

Cocaine production, more than that of any other drug, is a communal enterprise that involves the work and careful planning of dozens of individuals.

- After cultivating and harvesting his crop, the South American farmer sells his leaves to a local processing laboratory which refines them into cocaine. Frequently this lab is owned by the farmers communally, sometimes it has been set up by a local criminal enterprise.
- The cocaine is sold to a regional dealer who sells it on to a transnational bulk trafficker.
- A specialised shipping agent is contracted to move the consignment by land, sea or air to Mexico or the Caribbean.
- Another group ships the consignment across the frontier into the US to a domestic wholesaler. There are estimated to be 200–300 of these in the US.
- The bulk dealer sells onto a city middle dealer (estimated to be 6,000+ in US).

- Who sells to individual street dealers, who further adulter-
  ate and package the powder in single-grain wraps, which
  they retail to the consumer.

- Every step from coca-growing to selling on the streets of
  New York has potentially deadly ramifications for the individuals involved. Some lead such desperate lives that they
  have no choice in the matter. Others enjoy the thrill or are
  seduced by the money and, if they stay in the game too
  long, end up dead or in jail. The big winners aren't the coca
  farmers, who take home only 1.5 per cent of the profits, or
  even the traffickers, but mid-level US dealers who make 70
  per cent of the profits. This is first-world victory, where the
  West makes the most money and the producing and smuggling countries are left with bloodshed and environmental
  damage.

INDIGENOUS COCA RIGHTS

In 2006, the Bolivian people elected the first indigenous
President to represent them. Unlike his Spanish-looking
predecessors, Evo Morales, who is Aymaran, has dark skin
and features that resemble the average Bolivian's. His parents
were poor farmers and after starting off as a coca grower,
Morales joined the Cocalero union, serving as their secretary from 1985 to 1994. His role as a coca activist secured his
presidential bid by giving him a strong indigenous base which
supports his pro-coca and anti-American policies. Like his
two mentors, Hugo Chávez and Fidel Castro, Morales is a
nationalist and a socialist who wants to wrest his country free
of America's colonial yoke. Nothing, in his opinion, is more
representative of America's tyranny than its ban on coca.

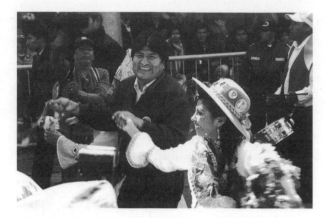

In April 2012, Morales caused quite a stir at the UN summit on drugs when he stood up in indigenous clothing and ate a coca leaf – reportedly smuggled from Bolivia to Austria in his book – in front of the assembly in order to make the point that the leaf itself is a harmless but vital part of indigenous culture. He and his coca lobbyists chant the phrase '*Coca Si, Cocaína No*' to clarify that leaf and powder are separate and that they are not advocating drug abuse.

Coca chewers do not need much to keep them satisfied and it is unlikely that many Bolivians are being deprived of leaves and consequently suffering from altitude sickness. Morales's spiel about the long-suffering coca chewers, although stirring, is not entirely plausible given that over 80 per cent of the country's coca leaves are turned into cocaine. Without wishing to question his sincerity, it seems relatively obvious that coca growers are primarily interested in making money. And money comes from cocaine, not coca tea.

Morales received a token victory in January 2013 when the UN, to the horror of US representatives, agreed to grant Bolivians the right to chew coca recreationally, thus overturning the UN's 1961 goal, set forth at the Single Convention, to eradicate the coca crop entirely. American diplomats still seem to have faith in the dream of a coca-free South America. This is never going to happen.

COCA-GROWING

The 'balloon effect' is a term used to describe the fact that drugs rarely go away for good, they merely change locations or switch hands – if you punch a balloon in one side, the air will move to the other. This is true of coca growing which, since the lapsed experiments in Java and Ceylon at the turn of the century, has been mostly confined to three countries: Bolivia, Peru and Colombia. When the coca supply is reduced in one country, the other countries pick up the slack.

Peruvians and Bolivians had historically grown coca leaves and sold the paste to the Colombians. But during the 1990s their harvests were devastated thanks to effective eradication policies, the closure of air transport routes and a coca fungus. Colombia reacted by growing more of the crop and by 2000 their share of the coca trade had swelled to 75 per cent of the total. America responded in kind and went after Colombian coca with a vengeance. Between 2001 and 2010, their fumigation policies decimated coca crops, and during those years Colombian coca production fell from 144,800 to 57,000 hectares. This led to a shortage of cocaine in America.

Coca-growing aggravates rural poverty and is disastrous for the environment. In order to avoid detection, Colombian growers push deeper and deeper into the Amazon, clearing large tracts of land and causing soil erosion as well as the destruction of biodiversity and wildlife. Poor soil is combated by dousing the plants with large quantities of pesticides, fertilisers and chemicals, which then enter the ecosystem in the form of toxic waste. The process of turning coca leaves into paste requires ammonia and sulphuric acid, which are also bad for the region.

One of America's key anti-drug strategies is crop fumigation. The rationale is that it is easier to destroy a crop at its source than to prevent the finished product from being smuggled. This tactic worked with opium but has proved more difficult with cocaine since it is tough and resilient and the chemicals affect the leaves but not the roots. Expensive fumigation campaigns have not halted coca production. Instead, the glyphosate and other herbicides which are sprayed on the coca leaves destroy other crops and enter the water supply, making people sick.

The poverty and lack of infrastructure in the coca-growing areas of Peru, Bolivia and Colombia is crippling. As mentioned earlier, coca growers make a pittance and the lion's share of the money is earned by American and European street dealers. Even so, coca-growing is often the only means of making 'good' money, since alternative crops like yucca and rubber do not fetch as much. Without other strong incentives, growers cannot be persuaded to halt cultivation, especially when their land is controlled by guerrillas and paramilitary groups.

COLOMBIA REVISITED

After the death of Pablo Escobar, the Colombian cocaine trade was controlled by the Cali cartel, led by the Orejuela brothers. By the late nineties, the Cali cartel had disbanded, giving way to hundreds of smaller, more fragmented outfits or *cartelitos*. The business was decentralised and fell into the hands of guerrilla and paramilitary groups. The age of big cartels and showy kingpins had ended in Colombia, only to be reborn in Mexico.

Colombia is regarded by some policy-makers as one of the few drug success stories and as a good model for cartel-damaged Mexico. Most of Colombia's dangerous traffickers were either killed or extradited by the late nineties, when the weak and fragile country became the largest recipient of foreign aid. In 2000 President Clinton launched Plan Colombia, a \$5 billion aid package aimed at reducing cocaine supplies and negotiating peace between armed rebels and the government.

Colombia is safer and more secure than it was during the cocaine wars of the eighties and nineties that killed hundreds of thousands of people and displaced millions from their homes. Murder and kidnapping rates are a fraction of what they used to be and, as noted earlier, coca cultivation is down. This is not reason to be overly optimistic. Corruption is rife, foreign aid is not always distributed honourably and the country is engaged in a three-way battle between guerrillas, paramilitaries and the military over cocaine.

Both guerrillas and paramilitaries are terrorist organisations with nominally political overtures that resort to brutal tactics such as kidnappings and crimes against humanity. The most famous guerrilla group, FARC, which still espouses Marxist/Leninist principles of land distribution, swelled from a ragged band of 3,000 men in 1985 to 20,000 in 2002, becoming the biggest insurgency in the world. American fumigation policies have helped push coca production into FARC's jungle territories.

Right-wing paramilitary groups – the most infamous is the AUC – are also heavily involved in the cocaine trade. They are notorious for weeding out 'undesirables' and for having strong links with businessmen, landowners and generals. Because of their military connections, American anti-drug money often ends up in their pockets.

MULES

Though the bulk of cocaine exports are handled by cartels or organised crime groups, there have always been a number of free-range entrepreneurs who operate by pimping mules. A mule, by definition, smuggles drugs in a body cavity – anus, stomach or whatever works.

Coke-filled body cavities make for good copy, which is why newspapers like the *Daily Mail* fill their pages with weird and graphic stories about hapless drug mules. One good example took place in 2011 when an Italian model returning from Brazil was arrested at Rome's Fiumicino airport. The reason the police questioned her was essentially Italian: she looked so sexy, with plump breasts and a great ass in a tight dress with cleavage. Both assets turned out to be implants containing 5.5 pounds of cocaine.

THAT'S A REAL DRUGS BUST!
WOMAN SEIZED AT AIRPORT WITH TWO BAGS OF COCAINE INSIDE HER BREASTS

Another similar incident in December 2012 involved a 28-year-old Panamanian woman who landed at the Barcelona airport and was busted in the wrong way. Her cocaine-stuffed breast implants burst in flight. Blood was streaming from her chest, coke had entered her bloodstream and police said she was acting funny. Almost 2 kilos of cocaine were removed from her breasts.

THE DRUG-MULE DOGS: ANIMALS FORCED TO SWALLOW BAGS OF COCAINE BY GANGS WHO THEN SLICE THEM OPEN AND LEAVE THEM FOR DEAD

Not content with human mules, who perhaps talk too much or expect a cut of the proceeds, some traffickers prefer animals. In 2013, Italian authorities busted a drug ring that forced large dogs – Great Danes, Labradors and mastiffs – to swallow multiple wraps of cocaine weighing about 3 pounds apiece. In order extract the drug, the poor beasts were sliced open with knives. Their bodies were dumped.

YOU'RE KNICK-ED! WOMEN CAUGHT SMUGGLING COCAINE WORTH £2M. . .IN THEIR PANTS

The Italians seem to be the most creative smugglers of them all. In 2010, they outdid themselves when it turned out that a convent outside of Milan was at the centre of a cocaine scandal. The nuns were blissfully unaware of the fact that some of the convent's employees were making pilgrimages to South America and coming back with cocaine in their prayer books.

COPS OBTAIN WARRANT TO SEARCH STATEN ISLAND SUSPECT'S BUTT; ALLEGEDLY FIND 41 COCAINE BAGS

While these ridiculous stories are potentially amusing in a sick sort of way, there is a dark side to a practice that is dangerous and exploitative. Capsules may rupture, killing you en route, or you may end up being killed or robbed by traffickers on arrival. Mothers are coerced or persuaded into making one 'easy' trip but end up getting caught and serving long sentences in foreign prisons while their offspring are raised by relatives. In 2002 alone, 400 Jamaican women (many of whom were mothers) were imprisoned in the UK for trying to smuggle cocaine.

Some mules have a great talent for ingesting cocaine. In November 2007, two London-based teenagers from Lithuania each managed to swallow eight condoms full of cocaine – about 4 kilos worth. Condoms are used because they are strong, lightweight and expandable. They are popular because they hold a lot of cocaine, but they also have a tendency to burst. This is usually fatal.

A lot can go wrong for mules and there are some standard procedures for how to ensure the safest possible journey given the circumstances. Grape-sized balls of cocaine are dipped in wax and wrapped three or four times in plastic. Constipation is encouraged, since every time you go to the bathroom you must wash the coke balls. This is the easy part. Then you have to get through customs.

In 2002 and 2007, the UK government launched two successful sting operations in cooperation with Jamaica and Ghana respectively, in order to cut down on air smuggling. The first, Operation Airbridge, was initiated after it was discovered that a whopping 25 per cent of passengers coming in from Jamaica were loaded up with cocaine. Although this book has devoted little coverage to Jamaica and the Caribbean, the region, which still provides America with 10 per cent of its cocaine, was terribly affected by the cocaine bonanza of the seventies and eighties, when it was the main smuggling port of entry in the US. Jamaica still has one of the highest murder rates in the world and a down-and-out economy. For people with no employment options, cocaine smuggling is worth the risk.

Operation Westbridge, the Ghanaian sting operation, deployed high-tech surveillance equipment and fluid tests to monitor flights between Accra and different European cities. The operation uncovered thirty-two drug mules on a single flight to Amsterdam. Statistics like this reveal the extent to which West Africa and Europe are becoming the new hubs of cocaine distribution and consumption. They also beg the question of how many mules are slipping through customs unnoticed.

Sting operations are expensive and time-consuming. And drug smugglers are endlessly adaptable, choosing different mules in different locations if familiar routes are being monitored too closely. As long as drugs are illegal, there will always be willing and unwilling mules to stumble uncomfortably through customs with crossed fingers and palpitating hearts.

PROFILE: LINDSAY SANDIFORD (1956—)

A common traveller's nightmare involves getting caught up in the Byzantine legal system of a foreign country over a cooked-up crime. In the case of Lindsay Sandiford, a 56-year-old retired legal secretary from Redcar, she ended up in jail for legitimate reasons: she was caught smuggling 4.8 kilograms of cocaine (worth £1.7 million) in a suitcase from Bangkok to Bali.

The international community (i.e. Britain and America) expressed outrage when the Indonesian judiciary system sentenced Sandiford to death by firing squad in January 2013. While charities like Reprieve bemoaned the inhumanity of this ruling, Sandifords's old neighbours took a more sanguine view of the affair. 'It's a shame but she shouldn't have been smuggling drugs and the law's the law,' they said.

Sandiford was not popular with her neighbours. In fact, she was the neighbour from hell. She 'wasn't a nice person' or even a 'normal housewife', they reported. And she had a knack for negative self-publicity, appearing in the local newspaper twice, once over an argument with the local council about her son, Eliot, and once over a broken Xbox. Her neighbours were pleased when she got evicted from her rented £275,000 property and went to India for good at the beginning of 2012.

Sandiford's Indian chapter started off promisingly and there are pictures of her grinning with red lips and a blue salwar kameez. But it wasn't long before she got mixed up with a small British drug ring in Thailand, where she and her new friends (Julian Ponder, 43, a retired antiques dealer from Brighton, his girlfriend Rachel Dougall, 39, and Paul Beales, 39) began hatching out the plan that landed Sandiford in jail.

Was Sandiford a vulnerable victim with a history of mental problems, as Reprieve suggests, or an idiotic but perfectly compos mentis schemer who wanted to make her fortune? She claims that she was coerced into the deal by her unsavoury associates, who were threatening her beloved Eliot, now twenty-one years old. They profess total innocence.

It is unclear why Sandiford's sentence is so much harsher than that of the purported ringleader of the gang, Julian Ponder, who was given only seven years in prison. The judge justified his ruling by saying that Sandiford's actions had hindered the government's efforts in their fight against drugs and had damaged the tourism trade.

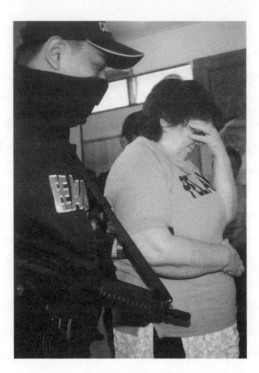

Indonesia is a foolish tourist's death trap, since cocaine
and heroin are cheap and readily available but the
country's drug laws are some of the most unforgiving
in the world – death sentences can be given for a few
grams of Class A drugs. There are 140 people on death
row – mostly for drug offences – at the moment and
about a third of them are foreigners. Indonesia has
no compunction about teaching hapless Westerners
a lesson and turning a hedonistic spring break into a
fifteen-year stint in Kerobokan Prison, a rat-infested
hellhole where you have to pay for your own food. This
is where Sandiford has been transferred.

Indonesia's death penalty regulations were outlined
in specific detail in 1964. If Sandiford fails to overturn

her sentence she will live off gruel in cramped living quarters until an unknown date when she will be awoken before dawn and ushered into a white van and driven to a quiet spot in the jungle or on the beach. Most prisoners choose to die standing but Sandiford will have the choice of lying down if she wishes. She will be permitted to take off her blindfold. The firing squad consists of ten to twenty men who have been given mental health training. Only two of the guns contain bullets and the rest are blanks. If Sandiford doesn't die after the first round, it will be the Commander's duty to shoot her in the temple.

Hopefully Lindsay Sandiford will be spared this awful death but this is looking increasingly unlikely now that her appeal has been rejected. She can still lobby the Supreme Court and then the Indonesian president but the process may take years.

The takeaway message from this sad story is that drug trafficking is no joke, especially if you are a well-fed Westerner with other employment prospects. American jails are awful but South American and Indonesian ones are far worse. And in the UK you won't be executed by the firing squad.

PROFILE: THOMAS MCFADDEN (1972–)

Thomas McFadden (pseudonym used in *Marching Powder*), a black Brit in his mid-twenties, who had been dealing since his teens, shouldn't have been caught smuggling cocaine out of La Paz's El Alto Airport. He was an expert in small-time trafficking and knew all the tricks of the trade – how to avoid looking suspicious (not by keeping a low profile), how to spot drug 'specialists', how to 'body pack' cocaine without poisoning himself and how to compress kilos of powder into thin plastic sheets which he covered in chilli powder to throw off cocaine-addicted sniffer dogs.

Thomas was very good but he was worried about America's War on Drugs in Bolivia, which had led to heightened airport security. He took the added precaution of bribing Colonel Lanza, a high-ranking police officer who introduced him to his children and promised to get his bags through customs. They would arrive at Charles de Gaulle airport in France where another bribed official would expedite the duplicate bag swap (see p. 69). Everything had been perfectly planned but Thomas was still nervous.

A traffic jam caused by *cocaleros* who were protesting American crop fumigation policies added to Thomas's jitters but it was too late to back out now. After checking his bags in without any glitches, he heaved a sigh of relief and walked over to the departure lounge. But just as he was about to board, he heard his name blaring out over the loudspeakers and was accosted by several policemen. They brought him directly into Colonel Lanza's private office, where he was greeted without any sign of recognition. 'The dogs have found something suspicious in your bag,' the Colonel told him coldly. Thomas McFadden had been set up.

Thomas was taken to the FELCN (Special Forces for the Fight against Drug Traffickers) headquarters where, after refusing to sign an admission of guilt, he was interrogated and starved for thirteen days until he was desperately ill and coughing up blood. Rather than wait for a court date, which could take months, he begged to be sent to jail, a request which was greeted with mirth but nonetheless granted. All Thomas's money had been confiscated so he couldn't afford the taxi fare or the 'entrance' fee to San Pedro, a prison where the state took a hands-off approach and inmates were expected to provide for themselves entirely, paying for their own food, medical care, electricity bills and accommodation.

Thomas couldn't afford medicine, food or a place to sleep, and after wandering around hopelessly had no choice but to collapse in the corner of a freezing cold courtyard and resign himself to his probable death. A Good Samaritan called Ricardo took pity on Thomas and took him to his own cell, where he nursed him back to health and taught him how to survive in San Pedro.

First off, Ricardo told Thomas that he had to master the sentence *'No soy Americano, soy Inglés'* so that gangs wouldn't attack him for being a hated American. Next he needed a source of income and, finally, he would have to purchase his own cell in one of the eight named and star-rated housing sections. Thomas learned that the rich lived in relative luxury, conducting 'business deals' and even leaving the premises on certain occasions, while the poor, many of whom were base addicts, lived in squalor. Base addicts were easy to spot because of their gaunt faces and desperate requests for money. Ricardo introduced him to an addicted feline lovingly referred to as 'Crack Cat'.

Cocaine was everywhere, in part because it was manufactured in makeshift labs operated out of prisoners' cells at night. Trained *cocineros*, or cooks, transformed the *pasta básica* into crystallised cocaine and could produce up to a kilo a night. Guards were paid to ignore the importation of requisite chemicals and the export of the potent finished product. Naturally, some of it stayed inside the prison and was readily available to the hard-partying inmates. Thomas got a job working in one of the labs, which paid badly but gave him unlimited supplies of cocaine.

Thomas gradually learnt the lie of the land by partying, fighting off his enemies and making friends in high places through bribery. Once he got the governor of San Pedro on side, his quality of life improved significantly. The governor, who was also an officer in the Bolivian army, shocked Thomas by showing up in his room with two giggling beauties before requesting 5 grams of cocaine and making jokes about gringo crop fumigation policies. Cocaine was tacitly accepted by everyone at San Pedro, which Thomas began alluding to as the 'International University of Cocaine'.

San Pedro housed several major drug traffickers including Barbachoca – 'Red Beard' – who had been caught flying 4.2 tons of cocaine, the biggest drug bust in Bolivian history. But everyone from big-time traffickers to minor dealers continued to conduct drug deals, which they referred to as *negotios*, from inside the prison. Thomas was in great demand because of his European contacts and managed to make $30,000 without doing anything other than providing a resident dealer with a good European buyer. He used this money to bribe judges and lawyers in his endlessly postponed court date.

Thomas had become a fully integrated member of the San Pedro community. He became the resident tour guide, bringing fee paying foreign tourists into the prison for coke-fuelled partying, conversation and a hint of danger. Thomas's fame spread throughout the tourist community of Bolivia until his unusual tours were even written up in the *Lonely Planet* guidebook.

After about three years of being incarcerated, Thomas's luck took a rapid turn for the worse. He was falsely accused of trafficking 200 grams of cocaine, an offence that could add a decade to his original sentence. Thomas was sent to La Grulla, a maximum-security prison where he and five others were locked up for twenty hours a day and subjected to physical and mental torture. At one point La Grulla received a special inmate in the form of Colonel Sanchez, an infamous politician who had embezzled $40 million from the Bolivian people.

Thomas was eventually taken back to San Pedro, which had been rocked by the tragedy of the rape and murder of a six-year-old girl. He kept a low profile for about a year but feared he might spend the rest of his life in a Bolivian jail. In order to pay for the inevitable

bribes that would accompany his next court appearance he resorted to mailing cocaine from prison to
outside customers who had placed orders via telephone
and email.

The trial was predictably corrupt and the judges
overseeing the court case agreed to set Thomas free for
$4,000 each, an amount he simply couldn't afford. With
the help of a plucky Australian backpacker called Rusty
Young, who had agreed to write a book about Thomas's
experience in jail, Thomas cobbled some of the money
together and then told the judges that he would pay the
rest upon release. Thomas knew that Bolivian bribes
didn't usually work that way and expected the worst.
To his amazement an innocent verdict was pronounced
and he was released from San Pedro prison on 28
December 2000 after four years and eight months in
jail. He managed to leave the country without paying
off the judges and promised himself that he would give
up his career as a drug trafficker and would never touch
cocaine again.

PROFILE: PAUL FRAMPTON (1943–)

Born in Worcestershire in 1943 to middle-class parents,
the young Paul Frampton excelled academically and
attended Brasenose College, Oxford, where he earned a
double first and went on to get his PhD. For many years
Frampton was a tenured professor of physics and astron-
omy at the University of North Carolina, publishing

papers on the phenomenology of particles and doing research for the US Department of Energy.

Not everyone at the university liked the absent-minded Brit, who was also startlingly arrogant. He gave a speech at a faculty member's 80th birthday party in which he repeatedly compared himself to Newton and bragged about being in the top 1 percentile of human intelligence. He also liked to calculate the probability of his earning a Nobel Prize.

Love was an afterthought for Frampton. He married a pleasant, middle-aged woman when he was fifty, but they divorced fifteen years later. He then set his sights on women between the ages of eighteen and thirty-five – childbearing years, he concluded – because he was ready to start a family. He consulted various bridal websites and found an appropriate Chinese prospect. She did not take. Mate1.com proved more fruitful and through it he found the love of his life, Denise Milani, a Czech bikini model with enormous natural breasts.

Milani was shy about meeting Frampton or speaking to him on the phone. Instead, they communicated via instant messenger. They had a strong verbal rapport and quickly fell in love. He thought they were the 'perfect couple' because her looks matched his intelligence. She said that he was the best thing that had happened in her 'cursed life'. Frampton dreamt of their life together in North Carolina – Milani would work as a Victoria's Secret model before getting pregnant. First they needed to meet. The opportunity came when Milani invited him to join her in La Paz, Bolivia, where she was doing a photo shoot.

The trip to Bolivia didn't go well because of Milani's heavy work schedule – she was called away to Brussels for another photo shoot before Frampton arrived. Milani was very apologetic and said she would make it up to him by flying him to Buenos Aires where he would catch a plane directly to Brussels. She also asked him to pick up a suitcase for her. It was nothing special but had sentimental value. Ever-obliging Frampton complied. He waited on the dark street in front of the hotel and was handed an empty, tattered bag by a Hispanic man. He filled it up with his own dirty laundry.

Frampton flew to Buenos Aires, expecting to receive an e-ticket from Milani. After waiting for thirty-six hours, he decided to cut his losses and go back home to North Carolina. If she really wanted the suitcase she would come to him, he thought. He checked in his luggage and was about to board when he heard his name called over the loudspeakers. He walked over benignly and was informed by the authorities that he was under arrest for smuggling 2 kilograms of cocaine. Despite his protestations of innocence, the flabbergasted old man was thrown into Villa Devoto jail.

During his trial, Frampton's defence argued that he suffers from 'a schizoid personality disorder that prevents him from making normal social connections and renders him unusually gullible'. His ex-wife agreed, referring to him as a 'naive fool'. The prosecutors did not dispute that he was gullible. But they did produce incriminating evidence suggesting that Frampton was aware that he was transporting cocaine, even if he was doing it out of genuine love for a woman who didn't really exist.

The prosecution unearthed text messages such as 'I'm worried about the sniffer dogs' and 'in Bolivia this is worth nothing, in Europe it's worth millions'. And they found a note calculating how much 2,000 grams of cocaine is worth in dollars. Frampton claimed that the suspicious texts were merely jokes and that the calculation was done out of idle curiosity after he was arrested. The judge was not convinced and on 20 November 2012, Frampton was found guilty and sentenced to four years and eight months in prison. He is living under house arrest and will probably be released by May 2014.

6

COCAINE TODAY: NEW HORIZONS

THE LONG GOODBYE

In Chapter 4 we discussed the end of America's love affair with cocaine. Freebasing and crack tarnished coke's image with squalid stories of crack dens and crack babies, and the young found other means of getting high.

Between 2006 and 2010, America experienced a cocaine shortage caused by coca eradication programmes in Colombia, large-scale seizures and Mexican drug violence. The shortage meant that prices spiked and in 2008 the product was only 51 per cent pure.

Even though US cocaine prices have stablised since 2008, it is doubtful that America's relationship with coke will ever again reach the lofty heights that it did in the 1980s. Today's 5 million coke users seem paltry in comparison to the 10.5 million who sampled the drug in 1982. And yet, America still consumes more coke than any other region – just about.

The worldwide drug market is relatively resilient despite international policing efforts. And the cocaine market, while slightly smaller than it was because of America's recent forbearance, is still quite healthy. There are roughly 13–19 million annual cocaine users, which is not much in comparison to the 200 million pot smokers but still beats ecstasy (although figures do vary) and is comparable to heroin.

Without the insatiable American nose, cocaine traffickers are looking elsewhere and finding small but promising markets throughout the world.

EMERGING MARKETS

Coca-growing regions have low rates of cocaine abuse. *Pasta básica* (basic paste) is smoked by men in the immediate vicinity of cocaine labs but is not a widespread habit. It is the growing middle classes in wealthier Latin American countries who are turning to cocaine for the same reasons that it became popular in America in the eighties. It is a sign of being rich and glamorous.

In the past, any cocaine in Central or South America was siphoned off shipments en route to the United States. Now Brazil, Chile and Argentina are specific smuggling destinations. Cocaine abuse is becoming a problem in Latin America's two economic powerhouses, Mexico and Brazil. Crack use is especially bad in Brazil and *cracolandias*, or crack lands, teeming with destitute addicts have sprung up in Rio de Janeiro and Sao Paulo.

There are small but growing cocaine markets in South-East Asia, Eastern Europe and West Africa. Australians and New Zealanders now consume more cocaine per head than anyone else in the world but their populations are relatively small. The real cocaine boom is in West Europe.

OUT OF AFRICA

Since 2005 West Africa has become an important player in the international movement of cocaine thanks to its largely unmonitored coastline.

Consignments concealed in hidden compartments cross the Atlantic in freighters. They are then transferred to small fishing vessels off the coast and brought to shore with relative ease – it is difficult to stop and search a ship in international waters.

Cocaine is also flown directly across the Atlantic in aircraft. In the last five years, several cocaine-laden planes headed for Africa have been intercepted by Latin American authorities. Others have crashed. In 2009, the charred remains of a Boeing 727 were discovered in Mali. It had come from Venezuela and was full of cocaine.

Sierra Leone, Senegal, Guinea-Bissau and Ghana are the West African countries favoured by traffickers, because, at roughly 10 degrees north in latitude, they are as close to Latin America as they can be. The coke usually passes through Niger or Mali and then through Egypt or Libya. Because these countries are all experiencing great political turmoil, smuggling is easy, and a significant portion of the proceeds are falling into the hands of Islamist extremists. Cocaine use amongst West Africans is on the rise.

EURO VISION

While the North American cocaine market has been steadily contracting, the European market has doubled since 1998 when there were only 2 million users. There are now

4.2 million users, which means that Europe has nearly caught up with the US.

Cocaine use in the UK soared between 1998 and 2008, with an accompanying jump in cocaine casualties. In 1996, only 1.5 per cent of 16-to-24-year-olds had tried the drug, but in 2009 6.6 per cent of that age group had. Numbers started levelling off in 2008 and 2009, perhaps because of the economic crisis, and the market is now stable rather than growing.

Cocaine is still very popular in Europe although it may get eclipsed by legal highs and synthetic drugs in a few years. The main points of entry into Europe are Portugal and Spain (either the south coast or north-west coast of Galicia) where 70 per cent of all European seizures take place. Shipments to Europe are mostly by sea and on industrial scale. Cocaine is also carried by mules on passenger flights.

Most cocaine headed for Europe ends up in Spain and the United Kingdom (Holland comes a distant third). Cocaine prices in Europe have halved since 1998 and have not been affected by Colombian shortages. Coke in the UK is especially cheap, selling for about £40 ($62) a gram as of 2013. Good prices do not reflect good quality since the drug is cut with fillers such as levamisole (used to cure worms in livestock) and benzocaine (a strong anaesthetic). Cocaine bought on the street is only 10–35 per cent pure, which is why it sometimes sells for as little as £20 per gram.

CURTIS 'THE COCK' WARREN

In 1997 Curtis Warren featured in the *Sunday Times* Rich List and by 2005 his fortune was estimated at £76 million.

Other better-placed though less respectable sources assessed it at four times that, at least. He was credited with having built this wealth from astute deals in property in the UK and elsewhere.

The *Sunday Times* was correct in describing him as an astute dealer, but in cocaine rather than in property. Later that year the police raided his home in Holland and found 400 kilos of it, along with 400,000 guilders and $600,000 in cash. Despite the fact that, at the time, merchant bankers and celebrity child molesters figured in the Rich List, Warren's profession was deemed unsuitable. Though his fortune remained intact, his name was dropped from future editions.

Born in 1963 in Toxteth, Liverpool, his father was a Norwegian sailor, his mother a shipyard boiler worker. Warren was recruited to crime when he was nine, as his size enabled him to climb through very small lavatory windows. By eleven he'd dropped out of school and participated in armed robberies. At twelve he stole his first car. After assaulting a policeman at seventeen, he went to Borstal then graduated to an adult jail, where he formed a network of connections which facilitated his subsequent career.

An internship as a nightclub bouncer – progressing to chief bouncer – enabled him to select which drug dealers could enter, allowing him to set up reliable supply-side distribution. In the late 1980s Warren went into partnership with established drug smuggler Brian Charrington. Together they flew to Colombia to forge a relationship with the Cali cartel. This was characterised by mutual respect and, in time, trust. Warren neither used drugs himself nor drank. He had a photographic memory. Telephone numbers and bank account details were carried in his head. Moreover he was discreet and took no particular pleasure in killing. He wore tracksuits not designer jeans, eschewed bling and fancy cars and did nothing to attract attention.

Subsequent international operations went well and profits were invested soundly in property. In 1993 he and Charrington successfully shifted a large quantity of Colombian coke concealed within lead ingots. However, a second similar shipment was intercepted. Warren, Charrington and a number of others were arrested. At the trial, Charrington was exposed as a police plant. Customs knew nothing of this and the case was dropped.

On leaving court Warren went out of his way to walk past the group of HM Customs witnesses, saying, 'I'm off to spend my £87 million from the first shipment and you can't fucking touch me.' The cocky remark may have been irresistible but it was a mistake. From then on they were out to nail him.

In England he was constantly watched and he relocated to the quiet provincial town of Sassenheim in Holland in 1995. There, from a modest house in a respectable street, he managed his worldwide business. Telephone conversations were always in code and key individuals referred to only by nickname: Twit and Twat, the Werewolf, the Vampire, the Egg in Legs.

In the autumn of 1998 Warren was charged with shipping large amounts of cocaine from Venezuela, where he owned a vineyard. There the drug was dissolved into wine in the same manner that Mariani had perfected a century before. The bottles were labelled in a reassuring but unshowy fashion as 12.5 per cent plonk and exported to Britain.

Chateau-bottled Le Cock tasted well on the gourmet palate with a bouquet containing the hint of grapes and honey and an exhilarating aftertaste. The wine could have done well in the supermarket but Warren chose to distil it back to powder, which was sold to customers with more esoteric tastes.

Warren's foray into the wine trade earned him a twelve-year stretch in Holland. While serving it he was assaulted by a Turkish prisoner. Warren knocked him down, kicked him four times in the head and killed him. For that he got an extra four years.

In 2005, having been labelled Interpol's 'most wanted criminal', he was charged with running an international drugs cartel from solitary in his Dutch prison cell. He appealed, won his case and came out in 2007.

Relocating to the quiet island of Jersey, Warren retired to an ageing middle-class golfing community to live on his widespread investments. But dullsville proved too much for him. A workaholic, he was recorded as having made 1,587 calls in a three-week period from public telephone boxes in Jersey and North Wales.

In 2007 he was arrested in St Helier and police came up with a proposition: that he plead guilty and receive eight years with no confiscation of assets. Warren turned down the deal and was found guilty. He currently shifts residence between several jails, as a number of contracts have been taken out on his life. His fortune is currently estimated at £185 million. In Toxteth, where he was born, amongst the most deprived and hopeless of Britain's slums, t-shirts and a poster of him are selling well. He is regarded as a local hero.

A FUNNY THING HAPPENED ON THE WAY TO THE FORUM

Sometimes an act is so horrifying that the only way to respond to it is by bursting into hysterical laughter. The shift from tragedy to farce occurred rapidly enough when the story broke in May 2011 that a Bulgarian vagrant had successfully beheaded a 60-year-old British grandmother at a supermarket in Los Christianos, a resort town on the Spanish island of Tenerife.

Because of the grisly nature of Jennifer Mills-Westley's random death, niggling questions kept popping up. How did 28-year-old Deyan Deyanov get away with brandishing a sword in the mid-morning daylight before plunging it into the neck of the unsuspecting retiree? And what happened during the five minutes it took Deyanov to silently hack through the muscle, cartilage and bone so that he could detach the head and rush out with it yelling, 'I am Christ reborn and I will bring fire of the Holy Spirit on you'? Was everyone watching in terror or were they too busy lingering over the chorizo to notice?

A few brave men jolted themselves out of their frozen state and tackled the madman to the pavement under a palm tree on Avenida Juan Carlos. They had to pry the dripping object out of his clenched hands because he refused to let go of his 'treasure'. When the wide-eyed Deyanov was taken into custody they tested him for drugs and found crack and LSD in his system. They also looked into his records and saw that that he had a well-documented record of criminality.

Deyanov's compatriots in Ruse, Bulgaria had been glad to see the end of the thieving drug-addict, who went on to inflict his problems on other European cities. He drifted into Cyprus, Edinburgh, Bradford and the north-east of Wales, getting into scraps with the law and occasionally being sectioned in psychiatric units. But no institution wanted to take this penniless, unlovable foreigner into their care for good, allowing him to slip through the cracks so long as he cleared out.

This is how Deyanov found himself in the land of lobster-red expats who have cobbled enough money together to live out their golden years in tipsy bliss. Our nightmare product of the European Union was not exactly welcomed with open arms by his neighbours, who accurately pegged him as 'disturbed' and 'intimidating'. Still, not every downcast weirdo turns into an executioner, and most of us choose to ignore that which is unpleasant.

Mills-Westley's daughters cherish the memory of their beloved mother, who, they are quick to point out, was much more than the woman now famous for being beheaded. They spoke of a 'catalogue of failings' that allowed a drug-addicted schizophrenic out on the streets. On 22 February 2013, Deyanov, who does not recollect the incident or even recognise himself in the CCTV footage, was sentenced to twenty years in a Spanish prison.

It was the schizophrenia rather than the crack that caused Deyanov to hear voices telling him that he was an angel of Christ. But drug abuse, mental illness and crime form a potent cocktail that is not well legislated for. Each problem exacerbates the others until it is impossible to disentangle them. It is entirely possible that Deyanov's crack addiction pushed him further over the edge and contributed to his deranged crime. And poor Mrs Mills-Westley, who was just in the wrong place at the wrong time, was one of addiction's proxy victims, proving that drugs do not only affect those who take them.

PROFILE: DANNIELLA WESTBROOK (1973—)

She became notorious as 'the girl with no nose'. On *The Jeremy Kyle Show* in 2012 she broke down and wept, revealing that she stole from her husband to fund her crack habit, was on drugs throughout her pregnancy and snorted cocaine in the delivery room while giving birth to her son.

Danniella was born in 1973 into an upwardly mobile lower-middle-class family in Essex, where both parents worked hard to upgrade their circumstances and status. 'I came from a very loving family,' Danniella explains. 'You know, 2.4 children with a Volvo.'

Her father had a one-man business as a carpet fitter and doubled as a taxi driver during slack periods. Her mother was a shop assistant.

She was offered her first modelling job at the age of seven, an ad for Weetabix. Then she was chosen to front Next's line in kids' clothes. Asda also wanted her for a campaign. Her face – cheeky, joyous and pretty, but not too pretty – was exactly right. She was impudent and sassy and radiated exuberant health. She was cast in a commercial for Coca-Cola, with its foreboding maxim: Things go better with Coke. At the tender age of fourteen, she would find they did.

The children at her state school did not appreciate Danniella's newfound fame. During playtime, a jealous girl had sheared off one of her golden plaits with scissors. 'I was distraught. I couldn't believe someone could be that nasty to me.' Her parents removed her and she enrolled in the Sylvia Young Theatre School in Central London, where other students at the time included Denise Van Outen and Dani Behr. She had little time for academic studies as her career continued to prosper. She made commercials and appeared in a children's soap, *Grange Hill.* 'And so at fourteen there I was, thinking I knew everything there was about life ... Looking back now I realise I was very naive. I had never been kissed and I didn't have a boyfriend, I had never drunk alcohol or tried a cigarette.'

She was out for the evening with her friend Claire at a pub in Essex. She looked a lot older than her years and there was no problem getting in. 'There was a boy I had seen before and fancied...' He was a broker in the City. After about ten minutes chatting he suggested they go out to his car, a two-door BMW. While they sat there talking he took out a CD, spilled some powder from a wrap and used a credit card to shape it into two lines on the disc. 'Want one?' he asked.

'I didn't want to lose face. I was desperate for him to like me...' Twenty minutes later in the bar she was flying, 'I felt confident and up for anything.' She'd never drunk before but by the end of the evening she'd got through two-thirds of a bottle of vodka and bought her first packet of cigarettes, Benson & Hedges.

> I didn't feel out of it, I felt great ... when I woke up in the morning I felt fine, I'd had one of the best nights of my life. I knew I wanted to do it again. It was the start of a love affair that would span the next thirteen years of my life.

Danniella says she wanted to be famous, something out of the ordinary. She wanted to walk down the street and for people to recognise her. At sixteen she was in the popular soap *EastEnders,* and they did. She was cast in a West End musical and appeared in a video for the band Queen. By the time she turned twenty-one she was spending £400 a day on coke.

At first it was once or twice in eight weeks: 'I never let it interfere with my work.' After a time, 'I'd think it quite normal to have a line at a party.' She was not using it during the day. Then it became three or four times a week, until 'I couldn't contemplate going out for the evening without it'.

Heavy use altered her personality. She experienced abrupt mood swings, and lack of sleep made her irritable and irrational. 'My relationship with the drug came before any man or boy I was involved with.' Sometimes she did as much as 5 grams a day. She was so thin you could see every rib and every bone in her spine.

In 1995 she went unwillingly into rehab, checking

out after one week. The year after, she became pregnant, discovering the fact only after breaking up with
the baby's father. She continued to drink and take coke
every day. When her son Kai was born she snorted the
drug during labour and immediately after delivery. 'I
needed it to survive.'

In 1998 Danniella married a despatch rider she met
while filling up her car. Eight months later she filed for
divorce. In January 1999 she was in bed trying to get to
sleep. Like all heavy users her nose was blocked. She
sniffed hard to clear it and felt and heard a 'crackle'.
Going to the mirror to check her appearance, she froze
in horror. The inside of her nose had gone and she had
no nostrils, only a hole. The septum had come away and
'was just hanging there'.

Within two years she'd remarried. Kevin Jenkins was
thirty-two and a successful self-made businessman. She
made two attempts at rehab but relapsed and instead
had reconstructive surgery. The day she was discharged
she restarted using. Within a couple of weeks her nose
collapsed again. Her husband hired a 23-stone minder
and put the two of them on a plane to Arizona. She spent
five weeks in the Cottonwood Clinic. She was desperate
and near to death when she checked in. This time she
really wanted to kick the habit and she did, though as
she says, 'You're never really cured of addiction, you're
only in recovery.'

Few of the profiles in this book close on a note of
hope. Happy endings are scarce, but Danniella's is
one of them. She joined Cocaine Anonymous, then

Narcotics Anonymous and Alcoholics Anonymous. She attended three meetings a week, she became a born-again Christian. All of these provided strands of strength. As did a caring husband and love for and from her son Kai. He'd been with her through the worst of times. Once as a toddler he'd shoved a chocolate bar in her mouth when she was having a cocaine convulsion. And when she asked him what he wanted for his birthday or Christmas, the answer was always the same: 'A nose for Mummy.'

COOL BRITANNIA: KEITH RICHARDS, KATE MOSS AND AMY WINEHOUSE

The English have perfected the art of being cool. The French are too pompous and the Americans are too earnest to bring it off. But in fair Albion, two national traits – sneering indifference and substance abuse – complement cool. The English have a pronounced capacity for alcohol and drugs. And happily for them, there is nothing more uncool than saying 'I don't drink' or 'I think I'll pass on the coke'.

The Rolling Stones were cool. And Keith Richards is still cool even though he is nearing seventy. The craggy-faced old pirate has imbibed so many hard drugs over the course of three decades that he ought to be dead. But there he is in fine fettle, twinkling and grinning and strumming his guitar like a mummified schoolboy. Although he finally gave up his long-term coke habit in 2006 after falling out of a tree, he still likes to boast about snorting his father's ashes with cocaine.

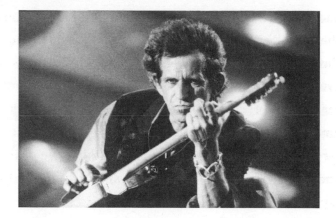

Kate Moss, to name another totem, has a strong instinct for self-preservation. Even if she smokes and sniffs and parties until her skin looks like sandpaper, she will never go off the rails entirely. She's too smart for that. And so what if she's starting to look rough around the edges? That's why we have airbrushing. As the quintessentially British anti-supermodel who brought in heroin chic and grunge in the nineties, she knows rude health is overrated, unoriginal and certainly not cool.

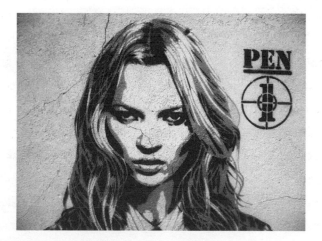

'Cocaine Kate' earned her moniker in September 2005 after the *Daily Mirror* plastered their front and inside pages with stills from a grainy video of Kate snorting cocaine during a Babyshambles recording gig. The video itself shows Kate meticulously cutting coke with a credit card while yammering to an off-camera friend. 'He tried to rape his sister. They put him in a home and then he did rape two girls. I've known him since he was six. Too much skunk,' she confides ominously and takes a deep snort.

Kate's baby-faced, drug-addict lover, Pete Doherty, blamed his manager for leaking the video for £150,000 which he spent on heroin. One might feel a twinge of pity for Kate, who, according to her defensive manager, never even wanted to be a celebrity. But then again, one might not. The fallout looked dire when she was dropped by Chanel, H&M and Burberry and was subject to a police investigation.

Complying with the requisite celebrity act of fleeting, public self-abnegation in the face of criticism, Kate broke her 'never complain, never explain' policy and issued a generic statement of contrition. 'I want to apologise to all the people I have let down because of my behaviour.' She vowed to 'stay positive' (as if that made any difference to anyone) and take the 'difficult yet necessary steps' to get her life on track (or had she just been caught red-handed?). Naturally, she checked into the Meadows Clinic in Arizona for a month or two and came back to England a clean woman.

In no time at all, Kate's career had recovered. Her income surged ahead of pre-scandal levels and in 2012 she ranked second on Forbes's list of highest-earning models. All press being good press, notoriety only added to her cool cachet.

Drugs don't damage your reputation as long as you can maintain your aura and your earnings. It's only when you start losing it like Amy Winehouse that you're in trouble.

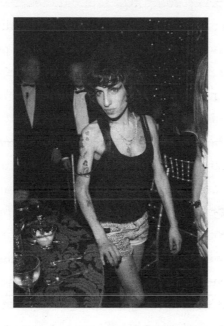

Poor Amy 'Wino' Winehouse – may she rest in peace – stands out as an example of how not to do drugs. She always felt too strongly to conform to the standard definition of cool. She adored jazz, Motown and the Ronettes, mimicking their beehive hairdos and swooping eyeliner. She worshipped her ever-present cabbie father, Mitch. She was head over heels, crazy in love with her toxic, soon-to-be husband Blake Fielder-Civil, the wrong 'un who introduced to her to heroin, which, in his words 'she took to like a duck to water'. She had always enjoyed pot but in her case the old slippery slope proved true; pot led to heroin which led to crack, the drug that destroyed Amy's voice.

Blake Fielder-Civil was happy to talk to the media about Amy's love of crack. 'The only thing she cared about was her crack pipe. We carried one with us all the time. If we went out to dinner, Amy would hide it under the table so she could have a quick hit,' he said. She would always smoke between songs and wouldn't continue unless she was high. While still only in her mid-twenties, Amy developed emphysema and an irregular heartbeat. According to Mitch Winehouse, her lungs were only operating at 70 per cent capacity and doctors warned her that she would eventually have to wear an oxygen mask if she continued smoking crack and cigarettes.

Amy's startling raw talent and original spirit accompanied her self-destructive urge. Her nosedive into addiction was almost as rapid as her meteoric rise to fame. Between 2006 and 2009, hardly a day went by without the tabloids publishing photographs of Amy stumbling barefoot out of clubs, Amy getting into fights, Amy covered in bruises and sores, Amy getting booed out of concerts for appearing drunk and high on stage, Amy looking anorexic and off her rocker and Amy madly frolicking in St Lucia in a failed attempt at detox. Some voices asked whether the world would sit back and laugh at her probable journey to death? Unfortunately, the answer proved to be yes.

PROFILE: DRUGGIE TOFFS

Being an English aristocrat has its distinct advantages. Hundreds of years of unearned social and economic affirmation have endowed them with a distinct sense of entitlement and they can bloody well do as they please, thank you very much. They disdain the petty regulations imposed on them by the small-minded clerk class – especially the fox hunting ban, the smoking ban and any law that reeks of puritanism. The toffs are a disarmingly hedonistic bunch.

The high proportion of aristocrats with substance abuse problems is not necessarily down to absent parents, inbreeding and a perverse desire to flout the law. A more prosaic explanation is that, just like celebrities and musicians, they can afford to be users and abusers – many aristos avoid nine-to-five jobs and still believe in full-time nannies.

Some of the best families in England form a lineage of addicts. Father is a drunk, mother is a pill head, Aunt Cleo drove off a cliff while stoned, Uncle Willie hanged himself in error. Getting a rise out of an aristo for shambolic, inebriated behaviour is not easy. It is teetotal Americans, intellectual pedants and people with dietary restrictions who raise their blood pressure. On rare occasions, an eldest son with no interest in beating his heroin habit will be disinherited in favour of a more suitable sibling. Sending the blackguard to rehab is a more forgiving option.

Rehab, that terrifying Gomorrah sung about by Amy Winehouse, can be quite pleasant if you have a big enough wallet. Clever capitalists cater to the rich's needs and desires by erecting drug rehabilitation centres in South Africa – people like to get away from the grim weather. The best packages combine health with holidaying and you are bound meet some like-minded souls from the right set.

If rehab is effective, you and Danniella Westbrook can continue expanding your address books at your next port of call: Alcoholics Anonymous (AA) and Narcotics Anonymous (NA). The Kensington and Chelsea branches, jam-packed with starlets, musicians and titled roués, are great for networking and sexual liaisons.

The Twelve-Step Programme emphasises the importance of 'total abstinence' and requires recovering addicts to invoke some nebulous higher power (not necessarily God) to ward off drugs. The format is confessional and heartfelt – everyone must share their own poor little rich girl/boy story which encourages intimacy. Besides, better to bore each other than everyone else.

Both drug abstinence and drug abuse are exclusive pursuits. Your refusal to partake of the drug is taken to be a judgement on users and a sign that you are not part of the club. Coke addicts are especially bad at admitting that they have a problem. Like Tallulah Bankhead, they think that although they use a lot of coke, they could give up if they wanted to. They just don't want to. 'Horses for courses,' the Honourable Celia will say when badgered on the subject. In other words, she is suited to cocaine even if others aren't.

Drug use may unite the classes to a certain extent but it does not promote social and economic awareness amongst the better-off. Does Celia worry about the Guatemalan mule who risked life and liberty transporting cocaine up her ass? Does she worry about torture and decapitation in Mexico? She does not.

Marx would say that we are alienated from the products we consume. We believe that objects spring into the world to be purchased and enjoyed and find it nearly impossible to associate a few lines of coke with a chain of human suffering. It is, therefore, pointless to think that people will stop taking drugs out of pity for the drug victims in producing and transporting countries. Our minds don't work that way.

UNHEALTHY BRITS

In order to avoid the accusation of toff bashing, we hasten to add that England is a nation of drunks and druggies. The country simply isn't health conscious. A UK health performance survey published in *The Lancet* medical journal in 2013 showed that while Brits are living longer than they used to, their quality of life is suffering and from about the age of sixty-eight they are beset by ill health.

Old Brits suffer more from debilitating diseases than most of their European counterparts. Despite high rates of smoking, Spain came out trumps because of their moderate Mediterranean diet. The UK, meanwhile, lagged behind in twelfth (out of nineteen countries surveyed), probably because of the processed meat, beer and crisps they are gorging on.

British youth, who are even worse than their elders, are a ticking time bomb for the NHS. Since 1990, when the last survey was conducted, drinking and drug using rates amongst the young climbed precipitously (figures have stabilised in recent years but the damage is done). Drugs and alcohol have been largely responsible for an increase in deaths amongst 20–54-year-olds. In 1990, drugs were the 32nd leading cause for young deaths and today they are 6th.

Statistics can be misleading and we should not take this to mean that the young are dying in droves from drugs. It merely shows that drug use amongst young Brits has become much more common in the last twenty years. Aristocratic Celia is not alone in her desire to imbibe stimulants. Middle-class students at Bristol, Leeds, Edinburgh and Oxbridge also take coke at weekends along with some MDMA. We are very influenced by our immediate circle of friends and if everyone around us drinks a bottle of wine a night, we are more likely to do the same. The same is true of drugs.

PROFILE: ALL THE WAY TO THE BANK

Cocaine and banking are both risk-taking, dopamine releasing activities. Very good bankers are gamblers who need to think outside the box in order to come up with new ways of making money. They need to be adventurous and confident while remaining alert and focused. They also like status. Cocaine is the perfect drug for them.

In the 1990s and 2000s, bankers reigned supreme in New York and London, and made the earnings of their eighties predecessors seem paltry. The Western world believed in their financial miracle without asking what it was founded on but demonised them after the economic crisis of 2007–8. Bankers say that they are scapegoats of a wider collective failing. The protestors of the Occupy movement disagree. To them, the world of Patrick Bateman in *American Psycho* has become a reality and the triumph of bankers represents everything that has gone wrong in a world of increasing income inequality.

New Labour opened London up to foreign capital in the nineties and helped transform the city into the happy hunting ground for the world's super-rich. Since the financial crisis, bankers are expected to look slightly more shamefaced about their conspicuous consumption. But there is a lot of money floating around and old habits die hard. Cocaine, which according to former drug czar David Nutt contributed to the financial crisis in the first place, is still prevalent in the milieu. Even if use is slightly down since its pre-crash heyday, it is now taken to assuage anxiety over whether they will lose their jobs or the bonuses that fund their lifestyles.

Blair, a Londoner in her late thirties, agreed to tell us her story about being married to a high-flying Australian banker. Blair, who does not come from a privileged background and is a career woman in her own right, settled into a house in Notting Hill with their children but never allowed the money to go to her head. She looked on the lives of her husband's colleagues with bemused horror. 'The bankers I met had all been inspired by the film *Wall Street*. They all wanted to be like Michael Douglas. I found that telling.'

When Blair and Ian went to Hong Kong she was struck

by how many of the top bankers were 'off their heads all the time' and couldn't function without cocaine. 'They need it to make deals because it gives them swagger. They start with a few lines to help them get through a pitch. If that goes well, they might have a few more for a reward. If it goes badly, they'll take it to feel better.' She says that they could get away with anything as long as they were earning.

A few years into her marriage, Blair noted that most of Ian's bosses were leading double lives. One, an old corporate broker, was married to an aristocrat and lived an outwardly respectable life in Knightsbridge. On Fridays, he brought out a little black book where he kept track of his brothel appointments along with the girls' names, abilities and measurements etc. Another boss married an intelligent banker but planted her into the countryside while he entertained his mistress in Chelsea. His wife became anorexic, started drinking and eventually killed herself by jumping off the roof of their house in front of their child.

Not all of the wives are miserable, of course. Many tacitly accept their husbands' philandering and party-ing as part of the bargain. Blair always thought that her husband was different from the rest and believed him when he expressed his strong disapproval of strip clubs and other sexist forms of 'client entertainment'. Perhaps he really did disapprove or maybe his objec-tions stemmed from guilt. Either way, she started to get suspicious and told him that she knew 'everything'. In truth, she knew very little.

Ian was relieved to be found out. He was cracking under the pressure of living a lie and told her to look at his laptop and his phone. She discovered that he was a coke addict, a binger rather than a daily user. He would do his best to stay off it for about four or five months and then go on a six-month binge. His main dealer drove a black Range Rover with tinted windows and they would meet near a tube stop, usually Oxford Circus. Ian would get into the car, collect his drugs (sometimes with an E tablet thrown in) and pay with cash or by bank transfer. According to Blair,

> coke is an attractive drug because it makes you feel bulletproof and special. You think that you can do things that ordinary people can't do. With a lot of coke, that risky side of your personality is nurtured and you start craving more thrills as you get desensitised to the drug.

Her husband's coke-induced thrill-seeking revolved around sex with escorts. Sometimes he saw escorts up to three or four times per week, occasionally during work hours. 'Bankers' minds are always spinning. They get bored or anxious and crave diversion,' Blair says.

Escort services such as 'City Flowers' cater specifically to bankers. They provide a high-quality selection of gorgeous young women, mostly under the age of twenty-five, who reflect the 'diversity of London'. Reading between the lines, any physical or racial preferences can be accommodated – not surprisingly, Eastern Europe is generously represented. Ian's tastes were different. He only wanted black and the blacker the better. Blair, who is mixed-race, attributes this to a sexual fantasy that combines power and strength with enslavement and domination. 'All the stereotypes are there in his head. Black women are hard work and can be kind of scary. There is something colonial about it, like a white master taking his pick of the slave women.'

Escorts can make thousands a night and are generally relatively well-educated young women. Bankers want a high-value product and won't be satisfied with any tart off the street. 'They are interested in ticking all of the boxes,' said Blair. 'In order to be successful they need to have a big house in the right area, a trophy wife, lovely children and a prostitute or mistress who is worthy of them.'

Ian is having a nervous breakdown and is in and out of the Priory, where he is being seen by a psychiatrist who deals primarily with City types. There is now a charity for drug-addicted bankers. Ian was promptly fired from his bank for a technicality when they realised that he was cracking up. 'They don't like mental weakness,' Blair explained.

> If you want to step off the treadmill, you are seen as a failure by your fellow bankers. It's far worse now that they are competing with nasty French bankers and workaholic American bankers as well as rich Arabs and Russians. You have much higher to climb and you can't settle for anything but the top.

There is a high burn-out rate in banking. Some drop out

relatively unscathed but others are ruined by the pressure and the drugs. Melvin Sabour, managing director of AKN Investments (worth $500 million), died of a cocaine-induced heart attack in front of his Mayfair flat in 2009. Darren Liddle, a 26-year-old trader at Credit Suisse, was another cocaine casualty. Darren, who had recently been released from the psychiatric hospital, committed suicide in 2008 by jumping off the nineteenth floor of the Park Lane Hilton Hotel after a cocaine binge.

Blair does not want her husband to end up dead and is nursing him through his crisis. 'He is drugged out of his eyeballs and just transferring addictions,' she says. He feels like a victim and blames the cocaine and the banking profession for his actions. Ian is begging her not to leave him, saying that Blair is the love of his life and that he will be lost without her. Other women might find these pleas compelling, but Blair has too much respect for that.

THE SILK ROAD

The internet changed how we buy books, music and other products. And in February 2011, with the launch of the Silk Road website, it changed how we buy drugs. Much like eBay or Amazon, Silk Road is a consumer-rated website where technologically adroit buyers – finding the site is tricky – can read reviews and look at photographs of products before clicking and ordering a few grams of high-purity cocaine from a dealer called 'Tim' based somewhere in California.

They can throw in a few tablets of MDMA and acid for good measure and await the arrival of a plain envelope delivered by the unsuspecting postal service.

Total anonymity on both sides is achieved with the help of Tor, software originally designed to protect the identities and locations of political activists in repressive regimes. Buyers and sellers are – for the time being – totally untraceable. The problem of registering credit cards or providing bank details is solved by using Bitcoins, a virtual 'cryptocurrency' named after the file-sharing program BitTorrent. Bitcoins are not regulated by any state but rather through computer programs on a 'peer-to-peer' basis. Initially, one Bitcoin was worth $30. Now, thanks to growing demand and economic uncertainty, each is worth $100 and the currency is valued at over $1 billion.

Even though prices are higher on Silk Road than they are on the street, this is a premium that users are willing to pay for quality control and safety. Advocates claim that they are keeping money away from drug cartels and criminals by purchasing their goods directly from more ethical sources, mostly in the US and Canada. They are bypassing the state and rejecting laws that they deem ineffective, particularly the criminalisation of drugs.

Not surprisingly, a high proportion of Silk Road supporters are libertarians and/or anarchists who believe that anything that is not harmful should be available to responsible adults. Drugs do not fall within their definition of 'harmful' but credit card fraud, weapons and child pornography do. The US government does not look favourably on this self-imposed code of conduct. New York senator Charles

Schumer has called for the website to be shut down and it is thought that the DEA is already on the case. Whether they have the intelligence to outsmart the computer programmers is another matter.

These are early days in the Wild West of online drug buying, but with the unpopularity of the War on Drugs and the difficulty of regulating the internet, it may be the wave of the future.

CONCLUSION

A few of the characters in this book seem to have possessed a wayward charm, others are tragic in their addicted life stories, while very many range from unsympathetic to villainous. We have mocked some of them for being hypocritical, spoilt, self-indulgent, deluded and plain nasty. We have also amply demonstrated the connection between wealth or fame and addiction. At the end of this anecdotal history, can we turn around and say that addiction is a disease rather than a wilful lapse of judgement and conclude that users need help rather than punishment? Might it not be better to let these reprobates stew in their own juices, either by locking them up or letting them self-destruct?

No matter how sarcastic your authors are, we don't actually take an eye-for-an-eye approach to drug control. And even if we did, we wouldn't want to continue punishing poor, developing countries for what is still primarily a Western vice. Without blaming America for everything, we have tried to show the devastating effects that the cocaine trade has had on thousands if not millions of people across the globe. Is this not an iniquity that we can amend?

The War on Drugs was declared by President Nixon in 1971. Today, more than forty years later, that same war drags on with mixed results. The DEA argue that they are winning and point to surveys which report a significant drop in figures since 1979 when drug use in America reached an all-time high. They see reduced coca supplies in Colombia and America's shrinking cocaine market as cause for celebration. Naysayers argue that drug use has shifted rather than decreased, as it always does according to the 'balloon effect'. They also complain that this pointless war costs American tax payers an astounding $40 billion a year.

Clearly, 'drugs' are bad for the health but are they any worse than alcohol and tobacco? Drug-related deaths (including legal drugs like sleeping pills) in the UK add up to about 2,600 per year and alcohol-related deaths are more than three times that. Smoking blows them both out of the water with 100,000 per year. There were 112 reported cocaine-related deaths in the UK in 2011, 393 deaths from antidepressants and 207 from paracetamol. (Why haven't we launched a war on paracetamol?)

The Netherlands has relatively lax drug laws. Their policy-makers believe that addiction turns into a public health issue when addicts contract HIV and Hepatitis C from dirty needles or die from a lack of quality control or from confusion over dosage. Nearby Sweden has much tougher drug policies but the two countries have similar rates of drug abuse, proving that harsh laws do not stop people using drugs. This was plainly shown in the 1920s with the failure of Prohibition.

Portugal is the most interesting case study. In 2001 the country declared personal possession of all drugs including cocaine, amphetamines, heroin and marijuana to be without criminal penalty. Despite dire predictions of the consequences, a survey by the Cato Institute in 2009 established that use of these drugs by teenagers had declined, the number of those receiving medical treatment had doubled, and the rate of HIV infection amongst users halved. Associated violence and criminal activity at street level had all but disappeared.

Portugal's model, where possession is legal but trafficking or dealing is not, is probably a more realistic solution than total legalisation. Still, the argument for legalisation is gaining momentum amongst a disparate collection of individuals including Latin American Presidents, libertarian ideologues, billionaires such as George Soros, and even amongst mainstream publications like *The Economist*.

In theory, legalisation is the obvious solution. The value of drugs would plummet and drug barons would lose their jobs. It would put a vast criminal network out of business and close off a key source of funding for terrorist and insurgent groups. Drugs would lose their illicit appeal. Addicts would no longer have to steal money for a fix. Quality and purity could be ensured and the health of consumers protected. The move would also significantly increase national tax revenue at a time of economic contraction.

In practice, legalisation would be very difficult to bring about. Over the past four decades the US government has built up an enormous narco-complex of bureaucrats, a whole army of federal employees. To disband these troops and put them on the labour market would not be welcomed.

Despite increased dialogue on the topic in the media, more voters in the US and the UK are in favour of prohibition. Proposing legalising drugs is too hot a potato for any politician. The move is guaranteed to lose votes and could ruin a career. The opponents of drugs – particularly in the US – are powerful and their moral position is entrenched.

Another sticking point is the difficulty of envisioning what legalisation would actually look like. Nightmare scenarios of crack being sold to children at convenience stores often shut down the discussion. Of course drugs would be regulated and licenced and barred from children. Of course very dangerous drugs like heroin would be strictly monitored. Of course there would still be a small black market, but it would be reduced.

Would a world where adults could legally bring cocaine to a dinner party, much like a bottle of wine, differ much from the one that we live in? Probably not. There would still be those who could take the drug in moderation and those who couldn't. There would still be addicts but the number of them would probably stay the same rather than surge. We are not policy-makers and the tone of this book is not intended to be didactic. But one thing is clear. Global drug policies are not working.

Since prehistory, mankind has sought for some substance that would enable an alternative and more cheerful reality. Should not individuals be free to choose the poison that best suits them? What follows to conclude this book is the brief record of a love story that says probably not. But it might not have made much of a difference in the case of Hans Rausing.

PROFILE: HANS RAUSING (1963–) AND EVA RAUSING (1964–2012)

In the first profile in this book Hans Rausing, owner of a fortune, who inhabited a rancid squat in a Belgravia townhouse worth £70 million, wrapped the body of his beloved wife Eva in several duvets and bundled her corpse into the linen closet. Returning to their bedroom, he shot up heroin and started a vigil over her decomposing body which would continue for two months.

It is possible to be exact about the date of Eva's death because of her pacemaker, fitted in 2006 due to heart damage from cocaine use. The normal heart rhythm is 60–70 beats per minute. On the day of her death there were nine episodes during which hers increased to between 180 and 384 beats per minute.

In the forensic examination of her body eight weeks later, following its discovery, it was established that its deliquescent organs contained traces of cocaine, opiates and amphetamines. Analysis of her hair found she had taken cocaine and heroin. Hans Rausing would be arrested for her murder.

‡

In his birth, his childhood and his adolescence Hans possessed every advantage that can be imagined: wealth, a stable family and unlimited promise. Born in 1963 in Sweden, son of one of the country's richest men, the billionaire founder of the Tetra Pak corporation. Hans was raised in his hometown in a comfortable but unshowy fashion. The family was not demonstrative and he and his two sisters were unused to displays of affection. Hans was a sensitive, clever but introverted boy and it was thought that the experience of private school in America would bring him out of his shell.

Perhaps that was a crucial mistake, but examining his life one is drawn to conclude that irrespective of his geographical or social circumstances, Hans was destined to meet his particular nemesis.

Withdrawn by nature, Hans didn't fit in at school. Nevertheless he experienced exhilaration in this escape from parental control and from the limitations of a provincial city. He got into weed and it suited him better than alcohol. He relaxed in the undemanding company of other pot smokers, where little was required of him.

The course of Hans's life from that moment on followed a classic trajectory. He dropped out of college to go to India and smoke dope on the hippy trail. He lived rough, as did his youthful fellow pilgrims treading the road to enlightenment. That goal eluded Hans though he did progress to stronger drugs.

He met his future wife, Eva, the daughter of a Pepsi executive, at an addiction clinic in the US. The couple moved to London in 1982 and by the date of her death had four children, aged between seven and twelve.

Mutual dependency bonded the couple, on drugs and on each other. Both shared a social conscience. Though they could not cure their own addiction, they could help others. They donated £100,000 to launch Mentor, an anti-drug organisation, and Eva served on the board of Action on Addiction, a well-regarded charity assisting young people with drink and drug problems. 'One very special philanthropist,' was how Prince Charles chose to describe Hans, who contributed generously to the Prince's Trust.

Eva's open and gregarious nature was different from her uncommunicative husband's. She could be lively and sociable, when in the mood. Hans was reclusive and socially inept. 'Vacant', 'monosyllabic' and 'blank' was how people described him. They went out seldom and attracted no press attention. They weren't interesting enough.

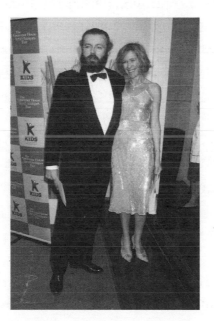

That perception changed dramatically in 2008 when the couple was invited to a reception at the US embassy.

The great and good would be there together with the elite community of charity patrons. Eva persuaded her reluctant husband they must attend. When suitably primed she could network and sparkle – but it took repeated visits to the powder room to replenish her vivacity.

When the car delivered the couple to the embassy Eva was carrying a vial of crack and a pipe in her handbag. It wasn't a wise move but cocaine perverts judgement.

At the entrance to the embassy all bags passed through a scanner. The shapes revealed in hers prompted a search. Next day the police paid a call on the Rausings' house. The bell went unanswered so they had to use a battering ram. Eva and Hans had locked themselves in the bathroom. When they smashed down its door Eva was alone with a plentiful stash of drugs. Hans had escaped out of the open window. Neither went to jail.

‡

Hans maintained his watch over Eva's body in the linen cupboard as May became June and a warm London summer. Even though its door's edges had been sealed and resealed with gaffer tape, the odour of putrefaction seeped out to taint the air.

When he required food – which was not often, for he was without appetite though gaunt from malnutrition – a tray would be left at the foot of the stairs and he'd scurry down to get it later. He'd told the staff Eva was in the USA.

June morphed into July. The hot weather continued. He was using heroin and sleeping pills, though even with drugs, sleep was hard to achieve. The only reason he ever left the house was to obtain money from the cash machine in Sloane Square and score drugs.

July became August, the weather remaining hot. On the 8th he needed to score again. To do so involved crossing the river to south London. It would have been wiser to take a taxi rather than his own car, but his thoughts and actions were no longer underpinned by reason. He was stopped in Clapham for erratic driving. Allowed to leave his vehicle and return home by taxi, police visited the house in Cadogan Place next day.

Even in the hall two flights below its source, the smell was recognisable, the nauseating miasma of death. The bundle in the linen closet and its rotting contents were exposed within minutes of the law's arrival.

Hans's vigil ended in his arrest for murder. Despite the initial charge, he pleaded guilty to preventing the lawful and decent burial of his wife and was given two suspended sentences. He is still in rehab.

In January 2012 Rausing walked out of the rehabilitation centre in Marylebone where he was confined, caught a taxi and checked into the Dorchester Hotel. It took two days for the police to trace him.

A NOTE ON THE SOURCES

BOOKS

Beith, Malcolm, *The Last Narco: Hunting El Chapo, the World's Most Wanted Drug Lord*, Penguin Books, 2010

Bogazianos, Dimitri A., *5 Grams: Crack Cocaine, Rap Music and the War on Drugs*, New York University Press, 2012

Bowden, Mark, *Killing Pablo: The Inside Story of the Manhunt for the Most Powerful Criminal in History*, Atlantic Books, 2001

Bret, David, *Tallulah Bankhead: A Scandalous Life*, Robson Books, 1996

Cooper, Edith Fairman, *The Emergence of Crack Cocaine Abuse*, Novinka Books, 2002

Easton Ellis, Bret, *American Psycho*, Vintage Contemporaries, 1991

Feiling, Tom, *The Candy Machine: How Cocaine Took Over the World*, Penguin Books, 2009

Foster, Olive M., *Crack (Drugs: The Straight Facts)*, Infobase Publishing, 2008

Fraser-Smith, C., *Lenny, Lefty and the Chancellor: The Len Bias Tragedy and the Search for Reform in Big-Time College Basketball*, Bancroft Press, 1992

Friesendorf, Cornelius, *US Foreign Policy and the War on Drugs: Displacing the Cocaine and Heroin Industry*, Routledge, 2007

Gootenberg, Paul (ed.), *Cocaine: Global Histories*, Routledge, 1999

Gordon, Mel, *The Seven Addictions and Five Professions of Anita Berber: Weimar Berlin's Priestess of Decadence*, Feral House, 2006

Grillo, Ioan, *El Narco: The Bloody Rise of Mexican Drug Cartels*, Bloomsbury, 2012

Grim, Ryan, *This is Your Country on Drugs: The Secret History of Getting High in America*, John Wiley & Sons Inc., 2009

Gugliotta, Guy and Leen, Jeff, *Kings of Cocaine: Inside the Medellín Cartel – An Astonishing True Story of Murder, Money, and International Corruption*, Simon & Schuster, 1989

Hoskyns, Barney, *Hotel California: The True-Life Adventures of Crosby, Stills, Nash, Young, Mitchell, Taylor, Browne, Ronstadt, Geffen, the Eagles, and Their Many Friends*, John Wiley & Sons, Inc., 2006

Inciardi, James A., Lockwood, Dorothy and Pottieger, Anne E., *Women and Crack-Cocaine*, Macmillan USA, 1993

Kohn, Marek, *Dope Girls: The Birth of the British Drug Underground*, Granta Books, 2001

Madge, Tim, *White Mischief: A Cultural History of Cocaine*, Mainstream Publishing, 2001

Markel, Howard, *An Anatomy of Addiction: Sigmund Freud, William Halsted, and the Miracle Drug Cocaine*, Vintage Books, 2011

McInerney, Jay, *Bright Lights, Big City*, Vintage Contemporaries, 1984

Sabbag, Robert, *Snow Blind: A Brief Career in the Cocaine Trade*, Canongate, 2010

St Aubyn, Edward, *Bad News*, William Heinemann, 1992

Streatfeild, Dominic, *Cocaine*, Virgin Books Ltd, 2007

Telfair Sharpe, Tanya, *Behind the Eight Ball: Sex for Crack Cocaine Exchange and Poor Black Women*, Haworth Press, 2006

Vulliamy, Ed, *Amexica: War Along the Borderline*, Vintage Books, 2011

Westbrook, Danniella, *The Other Side of Nowhere*, Hodder & Stoughton, 2006

Young, Rusty, *Marching Powder*, Pan Macmillan, 2003

REPORTS

UNODC: United Nations Office on Drugs and Crime, *World Drug Report 2012*, United Nations Publications 2013

UNODC: United Nations Office on Drugs and Crime, *Drug Trafficking as a Security Threat in West Africa*, 2008

NBER (the National Bureau of Economic Research): Working Paper 11218, *Measuring the Impact of Crack Cocaine*, Fryer, Roland G., Heaton, Paul S. and Murphy, Kevin M., May 2005

ARTICLES

'The Devils in the Diva' by Mark Seal, *Vanity Fair*, June 2012

'The Professor, the Bikini Model and the Suitcase Full of Trouble' by Maxine Swann, *New York Times Magazine*, 8 March 2013

'Cocaine Incorporated' by Patrick Radden Keefe, *New York Times Magazine*, 15 June 2012

ACKNOWLEDGEMENTS

Both authors would like to thank Sam Carter, Olivia Beattie and the entire Robson Press team.

ABOUT THE AUTHORS

Natalia Naish was born in Los Angeles to English parents and came to London after graduating from Harvard. She has a master's degree from UCL and now works for Bridget Riley. *Coke: The Biography* is her first book.

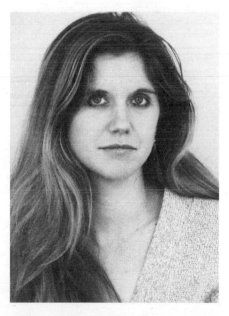

Photo courtesy of Alexandra Tommasini

After a colourful career in advertising, described in his acclaimed memoir *Fast and Louche*, Jeremy Scott became a full-time writer. His books include *Show Me a Hero*, an epic true tale of the air race to the North Pole and the historic deception at its heart, and *The Irresistible Mr Wrong*, the story of the ultimate playboy Porfirio Rubiroso and the innumerable women who fell under his spell. Both are available from Biteback Publishing and the Robson Press. He lives in London.

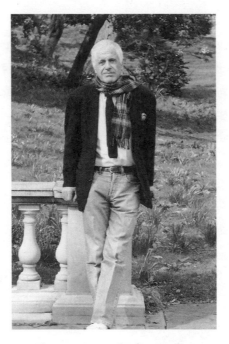

Photo courtesy of Jaime Brahms

PERMISSIONS AND PICTURE CREDITS

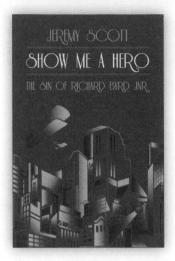

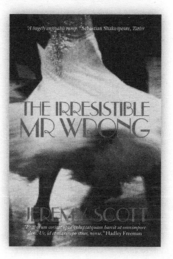